Kidney Dialysis and Transplants – the 'at your fingertips' guide

This book is dedicated to the late Professor John Walls,
who . . . just did it.

KIDNEY DIALYSIS AND TRANSPLANTS

The 'at your fingertips' guide

Dr Andy Stein MD, MRCP(UK)
Consultant Nephrologist and General Physician,
University Hospitals Coventry and Warwickshire NHS Trust

Janet Wild RGN
Clinical Education Manager, Baxter Healthcare Ltd,
Newbury, Berkshire

With **Juliet Auer** M.Phil, CQSW
Renal Patient Support Manager at the Oxford Kidney Unit

CLASS PUBLISHING • LONDON

Printing history
First published 2002

The author and the publishers welcome feedback from the users of this book. Please contact the publishers.
Class Publishing (London) Ltd,
Barb House, Barb Mews,
London W6 7PA
Telephone: 020 7371 2119
Fax: 020 7371 2878 [International + 44207]

A CIP catalogue record for this book is available from the British Library

ISBN 1 85959 046 2

Edited by Richenda Milton-Thompson and Sarah Brown

Typeset by Martin Bristow

Diagrams by David Woodroffe

Cartoons by Jane Taylor

Indexed by Valerie Elliston

Printed and bound in Finland by WS Bookwell, Juva

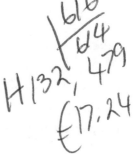

Contents

Acknowledgements

Kidney failure is about teamwork, so is publishing. This book would not have existed without the help of a large number of people.

Firstly, we would like to say a big thank you to Juliet Auer. Juliet is the renal patient support manager in Oxford; and, at our request, she 'took over' two vital chapters, 'Living with Kidney Failure' and 'Coping with Kidney Failure'. From the patient's perspective, these may be the most important chapters, but we didn't feel we knew enough to write them. Their inclusion is the major difference between this and our previous book, *Kidney Failure Explained*.

Many others helped with questions and answers on particular topics – either by writing them from scratch or by commenting and improving upon what we had shown them. So, thanks for this to the following people (in no particular order):

Rob Higgins (causes and effects); Gavin James and Helena Jackson (diet); Pauline Geiss (oral health and dentistry); Claire Morlidge (drugs and prescriptions); Anne Bakewell-Kuehnisch (peritoneal dialysis); Peter Ellis (haemodialysis and research); Nick West (living transplants); Margaret Peach (social and practical aspects); Althea Mahon (sex and fertility); Kate Craig and Anna Lynham (research); Monica Robb (useful addresses).

A group of Coventry patients helped to review the manuscript – Kenneth Payne, Simon Standley, Peter McGarry, and Jason Harries.

The book was reviewed by a combination of charitable bodies including the National Kidney Federation and the National Kidney Research Fund. We also benefited from reviews by the following health professionals: Terry Feest (the principal reviewer), Phil Dyer, Jane Harden, Cathy Holman, Richard Dingwall, Gillian Stein, Steve Nelson and Simon Wall.

The staff at Class Publishing (Richard Warner, Melissa Chapman, Emily Arbon, Judith Wise, Ron Haddon) were – as ever – patient, supportive and encouraging. They never pushed us harder than we could cope with. For this we are grateful.

Thanks too to Dave Woodroffe for the diagrams and to Jane Taylor for her imaginative cartoons.

Chris Denham, who is living with a kidney transplant, kindly agreed to appear on the front cover – along with his wife Sue, children Jessica and George, and Harvey the dog. Thanks to all of them.

There are four people who did above and beyond the call of duty. The quality of the book is not for us to comment on. But, we feel without these people, it would have been of much lesser quality.

First of all, we thank Juliet Auer (again) who did more than write two chapters – she affected the whole ethos of the book.

The text was proof-read by Andy's mother Gillian Stein (who also warrants a second mention), and one of the patients, Peter McGarry – to whom we will be eternally grateful. Quite how they spotted the 'the thes' and unnecessary 'thats', we do not know – even Microsoft cannot (yet) spot them reliably.

Finally, and most importantly, we would like to thank Richenda Milton-Thompson, our editor. She took over the job of editing the book from Sarah Brown (who got it off to a good start) and then raised the book to a level that we could not have achieved on our own. A book is only as good as its editor, and we had a very good one.

Andy Stein, Janet Wild

Foreword

When kidneys fail it is a major, life-changing event. The pattern of daily routine has to alter substantially, and permanently.

It is natural that anyone facing kidney failure (ESRF) should seek out information. Questions about the disease may arise one at a time, or they may arrive all at once in a rush. They may be asked by the patient himself or by other family members. After a very short while, the questions have usually become numerous and complex.

Medical staff in renal units try their best to offer advice and support, but they do not have the time necessary to explain the myriad of issues surrounding kidney failure. So it is all too easy for the patient to be left feeling frightened and ill-informed.

Because ESRF (end stage renal failure) is a rare condition, most doctors in general practice have little or no experience of it, and therefore are of little assistance when it comes to learning about kidney failure. Patients therefore turn to the Internet for information, to other patients and to books. This book is an absolute "must have" for all those with ESRF and for those who care for someone with kidney failure.

It is written in plain "no-nonsense" language, it is clear and concise. Above all, it empowers the patient with knowledge.

Timothy F Statham OBE
Chief Executive
National Kidney Federation (UK)

Foreword

Patients who develop kidney failure face a challenge for the rest of their lives. The miracle is that there are treatments which enable patients to live long and fulfilled lives after their kidneys have failed. The problem is that kidney failure cannot be corrected by a short course of tablets or an operation. Patients with kidney failure undergo a programme of dialysis, diet, drug treatment, social and psychological support. Even transplant patients need regular monitoring of their condition. Treatment is lifelong and complex, and has a major lasting impact on both patients and their families.

Life with kidney failure is a partnership between the patient and the kidney unit. The kidney unit can offer treatment and support. Patients must accept and use the treatments sensibly, and modify lifestyle appropriately, to enable the treatment to be most effective. It is unreasonable to expect patients to do this without help to understand their condition and the treatments on offer. The staff in the kidney unit try to help with this, but they are busy human beings, with ordinary human failings, and cannot do everything perfectly. It is hoped that this book will fill in some of the gaps, answer some of the commonly asked questions, and help patients to better understand kidney failure and its treatment. It should help patients take up the challenge of kidney failure, and use the treatments on offer to maximum advantage, thereby enabling them to live longer, healthier lives.

Terry Feest
Professor of Clinical Nephrology
Southmead Hospital, Bristol

xii

Introduction

Kidney failure is a family disease – it fundamentally affects the lives of patients themselves, and the lives of their family (which now includes the hospital team, their second family). This book is for the whole of this extended family. It is concerned with long term kidney failure, principally focusing on treatments, dialysis and kidney transplantation. It does not address the commoner, usually non-life threatening, kidney problems like infections and stones.

This is one of a series of books published by Class Publishing. The series is called 'At Your Fingertips' and its hallmark is the use of a question and answer format, giving clear and appropriate information in response to those questions you always wanted to ask your doctor. Class is a very small company based in Hammersmith, London. It has only a handful of permanent employees and is run by Richard Warner with the able assistance of Melissa Chapman. Richard is a dedicated, selfless and unassuming man who has an almost messianic drive to bring easy-to-read health information to ordinary people at a price they can afford. We feel privileged to have met him and to have the opportunity to help him with this mission, a mission we share. We hope we have kept up the high standards of this series.

Class published our first book, *Kidney Failure Explained*. The idea to write this one developed out of that relationship. Why write another book, if the first one is OK? Well, the first book was deliberately concise. In order to keep it short and snappy, we had to leave out some topics that we would like to have explored in more detail. Some of this material is included in Chapters 7, 8 and 9 in this book. It means that the two books complement each other more than they overlap. We wanted to be able to expand on some subjects – for example, living kidney transplantation. We also like writing!

We make no apologies to those people who might feel this book, like the last, is too 'hard hitting'. The chances are they would not be buying it anyway. If anything, it pulls even fewer punches than *Kidney Failure Explained*. But, in the wake of recent publicity about the National Health Service's failings, and about its future potential, we feel it is about time that the medical establishment 'came clean' on what it can do and, more importantly, what it cannot do. Its failings are not due only to the seriousness of disease or the technical limitations of treatment. Medical arrogance, poor organisation and 50 years of lack of investment in the NHS – for which we are all to blame – are unresolved problems.

We remain convinced that most patients and their families want to know the truth – no matter how grim – and they want to know it *now*. So that is what we have tried to give you. If you spot any mistakes, please let us know. Tell us too if you think there are questions we should have included but haven't. Repetition has been used deliberately, to drive home important points.

So, here it is . . .

1
Your kidneys and how they work

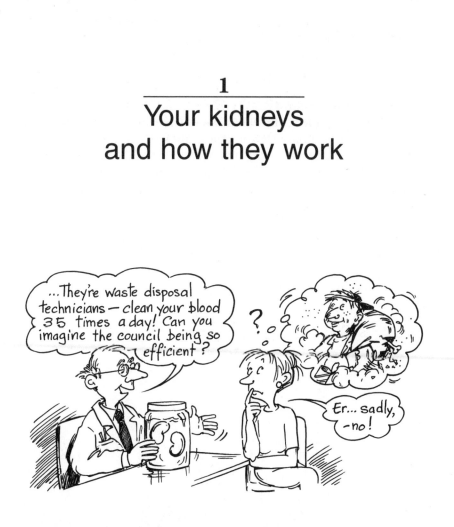

Kidneys perform many functions that are necessary for a healthy body. The most significant thing that they do is filter the blood to make urine. Urine is important because it removes toxic waste products from the body in a process known as clearance. It also enables the removal of excess water and salt. Healthy kidneys are extremely efficient, which is why most people can survive quite happily with just one.

Normal kidney function

What do kidneys look like, and where are they?

The kidneys are shaped rather like broad beans. They lie just below the level of the ribs at the back of the body, one either side of the spine – where they are protected from damage by the rib cage. They are roughly the same size as your clenched fist (about 12 cm long) and each weigh about 150 grams.

Why do we have two kidneys?

Most people are all born with two kidneys, although exactly why this is the case is not known. Many animals, including humans,

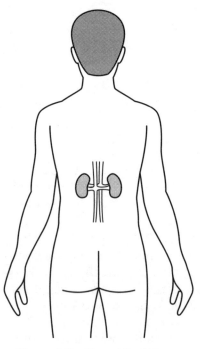

Figure 1 Position of the kidneys

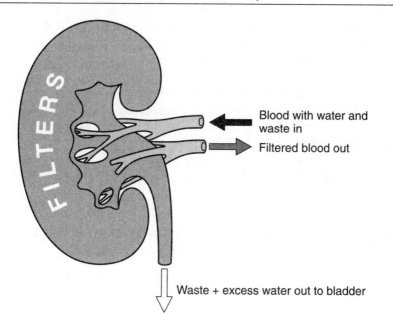

Blood with water and waste in

Filtered blood out

Waste + excess water out to bladder

Figure 2 The function of the normal kidney

have two identical organs, one on each side of the body. For example we have two lungs, two eyes and two ears. However, this is not the case for other vital organs such as the brain, the liver and the heart, of which we only have one. No one knows why we have two kidneys and only one liver. It is possible to survive on the function of just one kidney and indeed some people are born with just one. Many people have one kidney removed because it is diseased, or in order to donate it to a partner or relative. They can live very well without it, provided the remaining kidney does not also become diseased.

When I asked my doctor how the kidneys work, he said it would take too long to explain. Can you tell me simply how normal kidneys work?

Although the kidneys perform many functions, the most important thing they do is to filter the blood to make urine.

Waste and excess water are carried around the body in the blood. Blood from the body enters the kidneys via a blood vessel called the renal artery. The kidneys are made up of millions of tiny filters (glomeruli), in which waste products and water are separated out from the blood, to be collected and stored in the bladder as urine. The bladder can hold around 400 millilitres of urine. Most people pass around 2,000 millilitres (approximately four pints) of urine every day.

Adults of average weight have about five litres (10 pints) of blood in their bodies. All of this passes through the kidneys to be filtered about 35 times every day.

My doctor keeps going on about 'fluid balance', but I don't have a clue what this means. Can you explain?

The term fluid balance is used to express how much fluid is in the body compared to solids.

Balancing the amount of fluid in the body is a very important function of the kidneys, and one that healthy kidneys do automatically. For example, if you were to go into a pub and drink ten pints of lager, you would pass almost ten pints of urine. By the same token, if you don't drink anything all day long, you probably won't pass much urine at all.

When your kidneys stop working they also stop regulating your fluid balance, so this must be done by other means. There are two ways that you can control the amount of fluid in your body: by increasing or decreasing your fluid intake and by doing dialysis.

I know it sounds an obvious question, but why do the kidneys make urine, and what does it contain?

All food contains extras that our bodies don't need – and we usually drink much more liquid than our bodies do need. Urine includes the excess liquid and waste that must be removed from our bodies to keep us healthy.

Most of the wastes removed in the urine come from food. Salt and other small particles (such as potassium, bicarbonate, calcium and phosphate) that our body doesn't need are also removed. Larger solid waste passes from the body in the faeces. Although we need some of these substances, the wrong amount of any of them can be harmful. However, the kidney is able to work out how much to hang on to and how much should be removed.

Two important waste products are made by the body, rather like exhaust fumes produced by a car when petrol is being used. These are **creatinine** (made when we use our muscles) and **urea** (a leftover waste after we have eaten protein). Levels of these are easy to measure so they are useful as 'indicators' of how well the removal process is working.

Why do we need to remove water from the body? After all, it isn't poisonous.

Between 55 and 60% of your body is water. It is important to keep this amount balanced. Kidneys are good at controlling how much water there is in our bodies. You have probably noticed that if you drink a lot of liquid, you have to go to the toilet more often. Also, in hot weather when you sweat a lot, you tend not to pass urine quite so much.

If your kidneys cannot control the amount of water in the body, it will build up. This can cause swelling, particularly in the ankles (water is quite heavy and so sinks to the bottom of the body). In bad cases, the excess water can collect in the lungs and make it difficult to breathe. (See previous page for more information on fluid balance.)

What else do the kidneys do?

The kidneys have other jobs as well as removing waste, water and excess salts. In particular, they have three other important functions:

(i) they help to make red blood cells (the part of the blood that carries oxygen around the body);
(ii) they help to keep bones healthy;
(iii) they help to keep blood pressure under control.

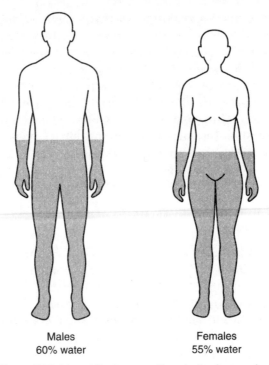

Males
60% water

Females
55% water

Figure 3 Fluid and flesh proportions in the human body

I'm a great believer in keeping fit and healthy. We are always being told what to do to minimise our chances of developing cancer. Are there similar precautions we can take to ensure our kidneys keep efficient and free from disease?

The most important thing you can do is to reduce your risk of developing non-insulin dependent diabetes, as this is one of the most common causes of kidney failure.

Diabetes is particularly common among certain groups of the population:

(i) people who are overweight;
(ii) people with a family history of the disease;
(iii) Black or Asian people.

If any of the above apply to you, or if you are over 40, it is worth asking your GP to have your blood and urine checked for excess sugar on an annual basis. If it is raised, you may have diabetes.

Together with smoking, obesity is also the cause of other serious health problems such as high blood pressure (itself thought to be a causative factor for kidney disease). So eat sensibly, avoiding fatty and sugary foods as well as too much salt, and don't take up smoking. If you smoke already, you should make a real effort to stop. Many health centres are now able to provide help and support with this, or you could try an alternative treatment such as acupuncture or hypnosis.

What can go wrong?

What can go wrong with my kidneys?

If they are to work properly, the kidneys need four things:

- (i) a supply of blood that needs to be filtered;
- (ii) filters to filter the blood;
- (iii) somewhere for the excess water and waste to go so it can be removed from the body;
- (iv) a way for the filtered blood to return to the rest of the body.

If any of these four are unable to work properly, the kidneys won't be able to make urine and remove waste and water from the body.

If the kidneys do not have a blood supply, there will be no blood entering them to be filtered.

If the kidneys do have a blood supply, and the blood gets into them but the filters don't work, the blood will leave the kidneys in exactly the same condition that it entered them – full of waste and water.

If blood can be filtered by the kidneys to make urine, but there is a block in the drainage system for the urine, the kidneys will eventually become swollen and blocked and unable to continue functioning.

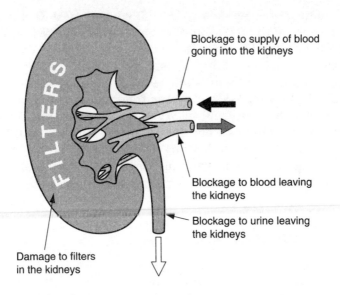

Figure 4 What can make the kidneys stop working?

Blood also needs to be circulated around the rest of the body once all the waste and excess water have been removed. This is important as it will allow purified blood to reach the rest of the tissues and more blood to flow into the kidneys for filtering.

I have always liked a lot of salt with my food. Now I am having trouble with my kidneys I have been told I must stop this. But is this really necessary?

It is certainly a good idea for most kidney patients to reduce their salt intake. This is partly because a high salt intake is thought to contribute to hypertension (high blood pressure), very common in kidney patients. Another reason for reducing salt intake is because salty foods will make you thirsty so you will have difficulty controlling your fluid intake. This will be particularly important if you start dialysis.

I get cystitis a lot and the doctor describes this as a 'recurrent urinary tract infection'. Is this causing long term damage to my kidneys?

Recurrent urinary tract infections are extremely common, in fact most women will have one or more such infections in the course of their life and some have them frequently. They can be very unpleasant but, in the vast majority of women, there is no damage to the kidneys. However, if the infections continue and you are worried, ask your GP to refer you to a nephrologist (kidney specialist).

My doctor says I have kidney failure, but I don't know what this means. Can you explain?

The term 'kidney failure' means the kidneys are becoming less able than normal to remove toxic waste and water from the body, control blood pressure, help to produce red blood cells and to keep the bones strong and healthy.

When kidney failure starts, it is likely to get worse in time. But this is not always the case, and it can take years, or even decades, to get to the point of requiring treatment.

When kidney failure is so far advanced that you would die without treatment (either by dialysis or a transplant), it is called End Stage Renal Failure (or ESRF). In this book, the phrase 'kidney failure' can be taken to mean ESRF.

What sort of people get kidney failure in the UK?

Kidney failure can happen to anyone, old or young, rich or poor. However, some people are more likely to get it than others.

Men are more likely to get kidney failure than women. In the UK, approximately 60% of new dialysis patients are male, and 40% female. This 60:40 mix is repeated all over the world. No one knows why this should be.

Black and Asian people are also more likely to get kidney failure than white people. This is also true in other parts of the world. In this country, about 6.5% of the population is Black or

Asian. However, the incidence of kidney failure in Black and Asian populations is at least three or four times that in the white population.

The reason that Black and Asian people get kidney failure is not known. It may be due to their increased chances of getting diabetes or having high blood pressure. It is very important therefore for young Black or Asian people to get their blood sugar and blood pressure checked regularly.

One of the main reasons people get diabetes is because they are overweight, so it is also important to keep your weight down – this is equally true for white people of course.

Older people are more likely to get kidney failure than younger people.

Most people who start dialysis in the UK are in their 60s, the average age being 63 years. However different renal units have different average ages. In some, the average age of people starting dialysis is as young as 55, whereas in others the average age is 71 years. This wide range is worrying, although there may be other reasons, such as a concentration of older people or people with diabetes living within a particular area. But, in theory at least, these differences might mean that older people in some areas may be less likely to be offered dialysis when they need it.

The number of older patients starting dialysis in the UK is increasing. In 1993, 37% of new patients were over 65 at the start of dialysis; 41% were over 65 years in 1995; and 46% were over 65 in 1998. This may reflect the fact that we now have 'an ageing population'.

Why is kidney failure more common in elderly people?

The probable reason older people are more likely to get kidney failure is, at least in part, because kidneys suffer wear and tear like any other organ in the body and get less efficient as time goes on. The kidney is made up of many thousands of tiny filters. When we are young we have far more kidney function than we need to keep healthy. One kidney can be lost without affecting health at all. Incredibly, half the function of your remaining kidney can be lost without you being aware that anything is wrong or feeling any ill effects. When we get older, this would not be the case, because the ageing kidney has already lost much of its 'excess capacity'. Any damage puts extra strain on the few remaining 'working' filters which are now trying to do it all on their own – and finally they cannot keep up with the workload.

I am 34 years old and I have been told I have mild kidney failure. Will it get worse and is there anything I can do to make it better?

'Mild kidney failure' is an ambiguous term because your doctor may mean a number of different things by it. A person with kidney disease could have mild renal impairment, moderate renal impairment, severe renal impairment or renal impairment that would lead to death without treatment such as dialysis or a transplant. In the early or 'mild' phases, many patients have no symptoms. Appropriate treatment of the disease at an early stage may stop it from progressing to later phases.

Unfortunately, many people with kidney disease will get worse in time. If their kidneys fail beyond a certain point, they will need renal replacement therapy (RRT). This will not be treatment for the disease as such, but rather a way of giving the patient substitute kidney function, either through dialysis (see Chapter 5) or by transplanting someone else's healthy kidney into their body (see Chapter 6). Some fortunate people may never need RRT. This may be because their disease has responded well to treatment in its early stages, or it may be because the progression of kidney failure is so slow that they die of other causes before it becomes too advanced.

When should I start treatment?

Every person is different, so the time when patients should start dialysis may vary. But there are two main reasons to start dialysis in a patient with kidney failure:

   (i) If the patient feels very unwell and has many of the
        symptoms of kidney failure.

(ii) If the levels of waste products or water reach dangerously high levels. One of the waste products, creatinine (see page 26), which can be measured in the blood, is the most reliable guide to the extent of your kidney failure. The blood creatinine level in people without kidney failure is between 70 and 120 micromoles per litre of blood. The higher the creatinine level, the worse the kidneys are working. There is no fixed level of creatinine at which people start dialysis, as other factors, such as age, sex and bodyweight will all have a bearing on their kidney function. However, as a rough guide, many people will start dialysis when their creatinine is somewhere in the region of 600 micromoles per litre of blood or more. At this stage, the kidneys are likely to have less than 5% of their function remaining.

I've got kidney failure and I'm worried about my children. Should they be tested for kidney disease?

Most types of kidney disease do not run in families. You will need to ask your doctor for details of your case. Generally speaking, some tests would be recommended if you have polycystic kidney disease or reflux nephropathy (see page 24), or if there is kidney failure in more than one member of your immediate family.

Can kidney failure be cured? And what are dialysis and transplants anyway?

Mild or moderate renal impairment, steps on the way towards kidney failure, can sometimes be stopped if it is diagnosed early and treated appropriately. However, there is no cure at the moment for end stage kidney failure. If you reach this stage, you will be given renal replacement therapy (RRT), in order to give back to your body the advantages of kidney function. RRT takes the form of either dialysis or transplantation. Neither of these are treatment for the disease process itself, rather they are ways of replacing the lost function of the diseased kidneys.

Dialysis is a treatment that can remove excess water and waste from the blood effectively and many people are able to carry on with normal life while undergoing this treatment. But if dialysis were to be stopped, the patient would probably not survive for more than a few weeks.

There are two types of dialysis – **peritoneal dialysis** (known as **PD**) and **haemodialysis**. More information about both of these is given in Chapter 5.

A kidney transplant performs all the functions of healthy kidneys, so is a more effective treatment than dialysis. However, transplants are not without their problems, which are discussed in more detail in Chapter 6.

Once you have been diagnosed as having end stage renal failure (ESRF), you will always have the condition whether you have a transplant or are on dialysis.

2
What happens when kidneys fail?

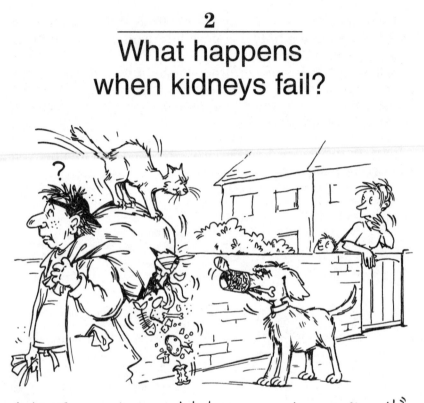

"Oh! These waste disposal technicians can be so inefficient!"

Kidneys can fail for a number of different reasons, and sometimes they fail for no reason that can be identified. Because the healthy kidney is such an efficient organ, by the time you start to experience the symptoms of failing kidneys, a great deal of damage may have already been done. This may mean that by the time your kidney disease is diagnosed, the damage could be irreversible. Even if this is the case, however, there may be steps patients can take to slow down the progression of disease.

What causes kidney failure?

I have been told my kidneys are failing. Why is this?

There are hundreds of causes of kidney failure, so we can't say what has caused yours. But you may well find it in the following list, as there are relatively few common causes. Most causes affect both kidneys.

- **Unknown cause** – doctors cannot find the cause in up to 30% of patients.

- **Diabetes** – too much sugar in the blood, due to under-activity in the pancreas gland – is the most common identified cause, accounting for around 15% of patients.

- **Glomerulonephritis (or 'nephritis')** – an inflammation of the glomeruli, the tiny filters in the kidney.

- **Polycystic kidney disease** – cysts (fluid-filled lumps) in the kidney, a disease that runs in families.

- **Reno-vascular disease** – slow furring up (and then blocking) of the arteries that supply blood to the kidneys.

- **Chronic pyelonephritis** – inflammation of the tissue around the glomeruli (filters), sometimes due to repeated infections in early childhood. (These should not be confused with the frequent urinary tract infections experienced by many women which, although unpleasant, are usually relatively harmless.)

- **Obstructive nephropathy** – blockage to the drainage system of the kidney, through which urine passes.

Why does my GP know so little about kidney failure?

Kidney failure is quite rare, affecting just one person in 2,000. Most GPs have about 2,000 patients on their books. It is likely, therefore, that you are the only kidney patient being looked after by your GP. Every patient diagnosed with kidney failure is referred to a specialist renal unit where they are cared for by experts. This means that some GPs get very little practical experience of looking after kidney patients.

Fortunately, access to the Internet has made information much more freely available to GPs. There have also been great advances in continuing education programmes for GPs in the UK, so many are becoming increasingly knowledgeable about kidney failure.

Are the causes of kidney failure different in older people?

No, not really, though many of the more common causes of kidney failure are more likely to affect older people. These include, for example, narrowing or 'furring-up' of the arteries supplying blood to the kidneys (reno-vascular disease). Another contributing factor is high blood pressure, which is also more common in middle and old age. High blood pressure puts extra strain on the kidneys and damages the filters. Some older people develop diabetes, which can lead to kidney failure.

Another cause may be a blockage somewhere in the system, between the kidneys themselves and the urethra, the tube where the urine passes out of the body. This prevents the free flow of urine and puts 'back-pressure' on the kidneys. The blockage may be due to pelvic cancer in women, or enlargement of the prostate gland in men. All these problems are more common in later life.

My doctor says he does not know why I have kidney failure, and that my kidneys are small. How can the doctor not know, and does it matter?

Unfortunately, many people with kidney failure don't find out they are ill until the kidneys are very damaged. As the kidneys become damaged, they shrivel up and reduce in size.

One way the doctor can find out what has caused your kidney failure is by taking a sample of the kidney (a biopsy) and looking at the tissue under a microscope. If the damage is severe, they will be too shrivelled to biopsy and the cause can never be found. But it really doesn't matter what has caused your kidneys to fail,

because the treatment for all types of kidney failure is the same –
dialysis or a transplant.

Will my kidneys have to be removed after I start dialysis?

Failed kidneys normally shrivel up gradually without causing any
pain or other problems. It is rare for kidneys to be removed after
someone has started dialysis. If you suffer from repeated urine
infections, however, it might be necessary to remove your
kidneys, especially if leaving the infected kidneys in place would
make a kidney transplant risky.

Occasionally, if you have very large polycystic kidneys (see
pages 19–20), they may be removed because they can cause pain.
They sometimes become so large that they have to be removed to
make space for a kidney transplant in the future.

**My doctor says my kidney failure is caused by glomerulo-
nephritis. What is this?**

Glomerulonephritis is the name for a group of diseases which
affect the kidney function. The **glomeruli** are the tiny filters in
the kidney. They are delicate structures and can easily be
damaged (see below).

Nephritis means inflammation in the kidney, so glomerulonephritis means inflammation of the glomeruli.

Some types of glomerulonephritis respond well to treatment
and failure of the kidneys can be slowed down or even, in some
cases, reversed.

The glomeruli are usually damaged by the body's own immune
(natural defence) system. The job of the immune system is to
fight invaders into the body. These might be germs or bugs, or
foreign objects such as splinters. The immune system is
powerful, and normally very good at recognising what is naturally
part of the body and what is not. But sometimes it makes a
mistake and attacks the body as if that part of the body was an
invader, causing inflammation. (For more information about
progression of disease in glomerulonephritis, see page 29.)

**Our mum is only 48 years old and we found out recently
that she has nephritis. It came as a real shock to us. So far
we know she has a creatinine level of 362, equal to about
25% kidney function. She has been told her kidneys will
deteriorate further, and she will need dialysis one day. Do
kidneys always get worse? Could this have been
prevented?**

Unfortunately, yes . . . kidneys, almost always, get worse. If there
is any chance for a doctor to reverse the kidney damage, and
improve the kidney function, it is usually at an earlier stage than
is the case with your mother. Say, when the creatinine is less than
200 (about 50% function).

Even then, treatments rarely repair *all* the damage, so that the
kidneys go back to normal. In those patients where a lot of
damage is reversed (say, to a creatinine of 150, equal to 75%
kidney function), the kidneys will usually deteriorate again, at
some stage in the future.

Doctors do not know:

   (i) why failing kidneys almost always get worse;
  (ii) why damage cannot easily be reversed, and kidneys then
       recover like other organs (such as the liver);
 (iii) why people with mild to moderate kidney failure almost
       always progress to complete kidney failure (called ESRF,
       see below) and require dialysis or a kidney transplant.

It is not all 'doom and gloom'. The following treatments may
delay the need for dialysis in some patients, perhaps including
your mother.

Treatments to control blood pressure
High blood pressure is known to speed up kidney failure. Doctors
therefore make great efforts to keep the blood pressure of their
kidney patients normal. Keeping the blood pressure really low
(consistently 130/80 or less) may delay the need for dialysis by
years. This is true for all patients with kidney failure – the cause
of the kidney failure makes no difference.

Treatments to suppress the immune system

When kidney failure is due to nephritis (as in your mother's case), the need for dialysis can sometimes be delayed by tablets called immunosuppressants. In some types of nephritis, the body's immune system (the system that normally fights infection or foreign objects in the body) starts to attack the patient's kidneys and stops them working properly. So, tablets that dampen down the immune system – such as the steroid called prednisolone – can be used to treat the kidney problem. In some patients, such treatments are very successful, and return the kidney function to near normal. In other patients, these tablets are less successful. Even so, they may delay the need for dialysis by many years.

Use of ACE inhibitors/angiotensin II antagonists

This is a more controversial treatment that may delay the need for dialysis in some patients. Some people with kidney failure (especially kidney failure caused by nephritis) have a large amount of protein in the urine. Normally there is hardly any protein in the urine. If a kidney patient has a raised level of protein in the urine, doctors often attempt to reduce it with a type of blood pressure tablet called an ACE inhibitor and/or an angiotensin II antagonist. Whether this treatment in fact delays the need to start dialysis (above and beyond their effect on lowering blood pressure) is unproven.

You should ask her doctor, whether there is a role for any of these treatments. If you ask your mother, you might find she is already on one or more of them.

I've been told I have polycystic kidneys? What does this mean?

There are several kidney diseases that cause cysts, polycystic disease being the most common.

Poly means 'lots of'. A cyst is a swelling with a very thin, clear wall, filled with watery fluid.

Cysts can be as big as a table tennis ball (4 centimetres across) or so small that they can only be seen clearly under the microscope. People with polycystic kidney disease (PKD) have hundreds of cysts in each kidney, and this causes the kidneys to get bigger. One or two cysts are common in people without kidney failure. Cysts may also occur in the liver and elsewhere. These are quite harmless and do not cause the patients to suffer from liver failure.

This disease runs in families. If you have it, any children you have will have a 50% chance of developing it too. This does not mean that all people with the disease should avoid having children as there are now very good treatments for PKD. (For more information about progression of disease in polycystic kidney disease, see page 30.)

I have polycystic kidney disease – why can't the cysts be removed?

People with polycystic kidney disease have hundreds of cysts. These cysts do not cause damage to the kidneys, rather they are signs of the damage that has already been done. Thus removing the cysts would not alter the function of the kidneys.

However, if individual cysts are very big and painful, or if they keep getting infected, they can sometimes be drained. This is usually done with a needle, some local anaesthetic to dull the pain, and an ultrasound machine (see page 85) to help the doctor find the cysts. When there a lot of cysts, draining a single one often doesn't cure the problem. If a person keeps getting bad infections, the whole kidney might need to be removed.

Do all people with diabetes have problems with their kidneys, and if so why?

Diabetes is a very common condition affecting 2% of the population (and 5% of Blacks and Asians). Around 40% of people with diabetes do have some degree of problem with their kidneys. The disease is caused by the failure of the pancreas to produce enough of a substance called insulin to control your blood sugar levels. As a result, the levels can go too high after meals, and too low if you don't eat. Sugar is needed for energy by all the tissues in the body.

If the levels of sugar go up and down often, it can affect some parts of the body including the kidneys, and long term damage can occur. Exactly what causes this is not known. The extra sugar in the blood of a patient with diabetes appears to act as a 'toxin', but there are high and low levels of other substances (insulin and growth hormone) too. So which one 'does the damage' is not clear – it may not even be a toxin or group of toxins. The high blood pressure suffered by most diabetics could be the culprit. It is possible that a combination of factors causes kidney failure (and other complications) in diabetes.

I've been told that my diabetes caused my kidneys to fail. How does the doctor know that?

Kidney failure can be diagnosed in people with diabetes by testing their blood and urine. Protein in the urine is usually the earliest sign of diabetes damaging your kidneys. The blood is tested for high levels of **creatinine** (see page 26). This can also diagnose the problem long before dialysis is needed, and before there are any symptoms obvious to you. (For more information about progression of disease in diabetes, see pages 30–31.)

My doctor says I have renal artery stenosis. What does this mean, and why does it occur?

Renal artery stenosis causes the main blood vessel running to the kidney to fur up and become blocked. This is also known as 'hardening' (leading to partial blockage) of the arteries or **arterio-sclerosis**. It usually affects both kidneys. It is a common cause of kidney failure in older people, especially those who have had a heart attack, a stroke or who have poor blood supply to their legs. These conditions are also caused by partial blockage of the arteries and, if you have one of them, it is more likely you will get another.

Arteriosclerosis develops in many of us as we get older. As well as becoming thicker and harder, the arteries develop fatty deposits in their walls, which can cause narrowing. Eating a lot of

132,479

fatty food, smoking, high blood pressure, diabetes and your genetic make-up may also contribute to arteriosclerosis.

When arteriosclerosis affects other parts of the body such as the heart or legs, widening of the partial blockage can be carried out using a technique called angioplasty. In renal artery stenosis, however, this is of value to a small minority of patients only.

It is important that all patients with arteriosclerosis stop smoking, lose weight, try to reduce their blood pressure and take a regular, small dose of aspirin as directed by their doctor. A tablet called a 'statin' (that can lower your cholesterol levels) may also help.

I've got angina, which gives me chest pain. My doctor says I've got renal artery stenosis, but there is no pain. Does this mean I haven't got serious kidney damage?

Normally, renal artery stenosis does not cause any symptoms. The arterial narrowing (see above) does not cause pain, and urine is passed normally. Therefore, the problem is only discovered when other tests are done – for example, routine blood tests to measure the kidney function.

Like many other causes of kidney failure, there can be a serious problem even when there are no symptoms. You may have badly damaged kidneys even if you don't have pain.

I have been told my renal artery stenosis will lead to kidney failure, and I will eventually need dialysis. But why can't it be treated with balloons and bypass surgery like heart disease?

Sometimes doctors try to widen the artery leading to the kidneys. The simplest way to do this is by placing a special very small balloon in the artery during an **angiogram** (see page 86). This balloon is then inflated so that the narrowing is stretched. This procedure is called an **angioplasty**.

However, even though the artery can be made wider, the function of the kidney does not always improve. Follow-up tests are also needed to ensure the narrowing does not come back.

There is a one in five chance that angioplasty can make the kidney disease worse.

It is possible for a surgeon to bypass the blockage using a piece of vein from the leg, but this is a risky procedure and in some cases will make the kidneys worse.

Whether any of these procedures can delay the need for dialysis is not known. There is no definite evidence that they can.

What else can I do to try to stop my renal artery stenosis from causing kidney failure?

There are several things you can do which may help the arteries to your kidneys, and any other arteries in your body affected by arteriosclerosis.

  (i) **Stop smoking.** Smoking also furs up the arteries and compounds the problem.
 (ii) **Eat a healthy diet.** Avoid fatty foods and added salt – ask your dietitian for advice.
(iii) **Monitor cholesterol.** The level of cholesterol (fat in the blood) should be measured. If this is too high despite a good diet, you may need to take extra drugs to lower the level.
 (iv) **Take aspirin.** Some of the problems in renal artery stenosis are due to tiny blood clots. Taking a small aspirin tablet daily reduces the tendency for this to happen.
  (v) **Exercise regularly.** Regular moderate exercise will be good for you, but be sure to discuss this with your doctor first in case you also have heart disease.
 (vi) **Keep your blood pressure low.** High blood pressure will continue to damage your kidneys and put strain on the heart and other blood vessels. Your doctor should measure your blood pressure regularly and may prescribe drugs to bring it down.

None of these steps is guaranteed to stop the kidneys failing. But they may slow down the process considerably, especially if you can achieve them all.

I've had a prostate operation that has made me pass urine normally after years of problems. However, I have now been told I may need to go on dialysis because it has caused a kidney problem. Is there anything that can be done to prevent this from happening?

Only men have a prostate gland. It is located underneath the bladder and usually gets bigger with age. This can make passing urine difficult. It can cause people to have to rush to pass urine in a hurry, or get up to pass urine at night. Symptoms like this often make men go to the doctor, so the enlarged prostate problem can be dealt with by an operation at an early stage.

Occasionally, the symptoms are not noticeable, and the large prostate causes back pressure of urine into the kidneys. This causes kidney damage. Although the back pressure can be treated with surgery, sometimes the kidney damage is so severe it cannot recover.

If you have had prostate trouble in the past and you are now developing kidney failure, it is important to make sure the prostate has not grown back and caused further back pressure on the kidneys. If it has grown back, another operation might prevent kidney failure, but in some people too much damage has already been done, making kidney failure inevitable.

Some doctors say I've got reflux nephropathy and others say I've got pyelonephritis. Are these two separate diseases, and will I get kidney failure?

Chronic pyelonephritis is a vague term applied to many patients. It can be applied to patients when all other causes of kidney disease have been excluded. It is presumed that chronic pyelonephritis is related to recurrent infections of the kidney. However this is often difficult to prove, bringing into doubt the idea that recurrent infections cause chronic pyelonephritis.

There is more evidence that reflux nephropathy exists. The theory goes like this. Reflux nephropathy describes the passage of urine back up the drainage tubes from the bladder towards the kidneys. This causes infections in the kidneys, especially in babies. Often these infections are very mild and are not noticed because they don't cause any symptoms. It is only later on in life that the damage caused by the infections is noticeable and kidney failure occurs. Proving this theory is more difficult. It is known for certain, however, that reflux nephropathy is more common in girls than boys and sometimes runs in families.

Only a few people with reflux nephropathy ever develop kidney failure, but once the kidneys reach a certain level of damage, failure becomes inevitable.

If you have a lot of urine infections even after starting dialysis, it may be necessary to remove your kidneys before or after a transplant.

I've got spina bifida and I'm in a wheelchair. I've had a lot of kidney infections because my bladder doesn't work properly. If I develop kidney failure, can I receive dialysis or a transplant?

Spina bifida can damage the nerves to the bladder so that urine is not passed normally. Sometimes this can lead to infections and serious kidney damage. Some people with spina bifida may have the urine in their bladder drained regularly with special tubes called urinary catheters and this may prevent infections. However, kidney failure may still occur.

Being in a wheelchair would not stop you being given dialysis, but may make treatment with peritoneal dialysis difficult (see page 93). Haemodialysis may therefore be preferred.

A transplant may be possible. However, to have a transplant you would need to be very fit and have a healthy heart and lungs. You may also need to have an operation to create an artificial bladder under your skin. An artificial bladder is made by a surgeon, usually out of a piece of your bowel that is reshaped for its new purpose.

I have high blood pressure and have been on haemo-dialysis for about a year. Is high blood pressure the cause of my kidney failure?

Most people with kidney failure have high blood pressure and this is often caused by kidney failure.

High blood pressure can cause kidney failure, but this is rare.

Progression of kidney disease

My doctor says my creatinine level shows my kidney function to be about '10% of normal'. How does he know this? I feel fine, by the way. My last creatinine level was 489.

When chronic kidney failure is still at an early stage, most patients feel quite well. This is because their failing kidneys 'overwork' to keep the levels of body wastes normal. This hides the fact that the kidneys are failing. In other words, the kidneys have a lot 'in reserve'. The body manages for quite some time to adapt to high levels of toxins and water in the blood. It does this by making the kidneys work harder.

To measure kidney function, we rely on a very important test – the level of a substance (that comes from muscles) called creatinine. It is the single most important piece of information that a kidney doctor or nurse needs to look after you. Its normal level is 70–120 micromoles (this is a very small amount of the substance) of creatinine per litre of blood. If you are reading this book, you should know what your creatinine level is – or that of your friend, partner or relative (whoever has the disease) – at all times. If you don't know, ask your doctor.

If the creatinine level in the blood is over 120 micromoles per litre of blood, your kidneys are not working normally. The point at which kidney failure is diagnosed will also depend on other factors such as how unwell you feel.

But, what does a creatinine of 489 mean?

Creatinine is measured in micromoles per litre of blood, so a creatinine of 489 means you have 489 micromoles of creatinine for every litre of your blood. Most adults have around 10 litres of blood in their body, but this will vary according to age and weight.

For most people with kidney failure, the following description will apply:

(i) When kidney function is 75% of normal, the blood creatinine may be 150 micromoles per litre, and you will feel fine.

(ii) When kidney function is 50% of normal, the blood creatinine may be 200 micromoles per litre, and you will feel fine.

(iii) When kidney function is 25% of normal, the blood creatinine may be 350 micromoles per litre. Even though you may still feel well, other problems (anaemia, see page 50; renal bone disease, see page 51) may have started to affect you, at least according to your blood tests.

(iv) You will start to feel unwell when your kidney function is down to about 10% of normal, and your blood creatinine is about 500 micromoles per litre. In other words, the kidneys have to get quite bad before you notice anything. For what you will notice, see page 47.

(v) When your kidney function is down to about 5% of normal, the blood creatinine may be 600–800 micromoles per litre, and you will feel very unwell. Dialysis or a transplant is then needed though, ideally, treatment should be started well before this time.

The symptoms patients get when they have similar levels of kidney function can vary considerably. Some patients get symptoms when their kidney function is 90% of normal, whereas others do not get symptoms until their kidney function is down to 1%. We don't really know why this should be the case.

I am a 78-year-old lady. My doctor says I have early 'mild kidney failure' with a creatinine level of 156, equivalent to 75% kidney function, and this is 'OK'. When I ask him what will happen, he says 'Don't worry about it dear, I'll let you know if it ever becomes a problem'. I wish he'd talk straight. Can you tell me what is going on?

The term 'mild kidney failure' is not strictly accurate. If you have kidney failure, the chances are that your kidneys will eventually stop working, if you live long enough. However, if your kidneys start to deteriorate late in your life, and they decline slowly, you may live out your natural lifespan without actually experiencing any problems from your kidneys. You may die of something different, in five, ten or fifteen years time, when your kidney function is still between 25 and 50% of normal. So, your doctor may be telling the truth, but in a patronising, and less than open way. You may die *with* kidney failure, rather than *of* it.

My creatinine level was 140 in March and 160 now (September). Does this mean my kidneys are declining? How does the doctor know how fast my kidney failure is progressing? I am a very busy person and want to know the date I will start dialysis.

The rate at which kidney failure worsens varies from patient to patient. The doctor will get an idea of how fast your kidneys are failing, by looking at the creatinine level in the blood, and the amount it rises from one clinic appointment to another.

So, for example, if your creatinine is 160 (about 75% kidney function) now, and 140 six months ago (still about 75% function), it would be difficult to say anything. The creatinine test is not that reliable, and a number can really mean any figure within 10 (higher or lower) of that number. So, 140 could mean anything from 130 to 150, and 160 could mean 150–170. So for you, both 140 and 160 could be 'the same' number (ie, 150), and the same level of kidney function (75%). Or, it could mean a real change, say from 80% to 70%.

In this situation no doctor could conclude absolutely that your kidneys had declined, let alone predict the date of starting dialysis.

If the 'jump' was more obvious – say, from a creatinine of 150 (75%) to 200 (50%) – this would be evidence of a real decline. The doctor could give you a (vague) prediction of when you will need dialysis. Even then, the prediction would need to be plus or minus at least a year. So 'you will need dialysis in about two years time', could mean you will need it anytime between one and three years' time. Predicting the start of dialysis is a very imprecise science.

I have glomerulonephritis, and the doctor tells me it will cause my kidneys to fail completely in about a year's time. Why can't this be prevented?

Many forms of glomerulonephritis do not respond to any known treatment. However, some forms can be caused by your immune system attacking your kidneys. If this is the case, it may be possible that certain drugs (for example, steroids) that calm down the activity of the immune system, will be able to reverse this process or stop more damage occurring. If the doctor thinks your particular form of the disease will respond to treatment you may be given drugs, but these sometimes have unpleasant side effects.

It should be remembered that all kidney diseases, not just glomerulonephritis, affect the kidney function. In addition, most causes of kidney failure damage the kidneys over a very long period of time. This usually means the effects are permanent. Once the kidneys have been damaged beyond a certain point, it is rare for them to recover even if further deterioration can be lessened. In most patients, the most effective way of slowing down the damage to your kidneys is by controlling your blood pressure (a type of blood pressure tablet called an **ACE inhibitor** is thought to be especially effective). This is the best that can be done to take strain off the kidneys and help them last longer.

My Dad had polycystic kidney disease and went onto dialysis when he was 50 years old. I have been told I also have the disease – will I need to start dialysis soon? I am 42.

Polycystic kidney disease is a common cause of kidney failure, but not everyone with polycystic disease will need dialysis. It does run in families, but it is not possible to predict if yours will need dialysis although there is a lot of research going on into genetic testing. In the future, genetic tests may help to predict your chances of needing dialysis.

In some families, it is very difficult to predict when you will need dialysis, if at all. It may be helpful to look at what has happened in your family over the years as polycystic disease often runs 'true'. That is, if everyone with polycystic disease in your family has needed to start on dialysis at about 50 years of age, the chances are you will too. If several members of your family are aged 70 and have good kidney function despite polycystic kidneys, there is every likelihood you will do well yourself.

I've been told I have diabetic kidney disease. Does this mean I will eventually need dialysis? Is there anything I can do to stop it, or at least delay it a bit?

It is true that diabetes can cause damage to the kidneys, leading to kidney failure. But by the time this happens, the diabetes is likely to have damaged other parts of your body too. You may have an increased chance of it also affecting your heart, your eyes, and the blood supply to your limbs and your brain.

These complications – including kidney failure – tend to occur in about one in every three people with diabetes, particularly those who have had diabetes for ten years or more. No one knows why only some diabetics get the more serious complications, and others don't. But there do seem to be unlucky people who get most of the serious complications of diabetes which others may be spared. There could be genetic factors at work, we don't yet know.

If diabetes has started to affect your kidneys, it is likely you will need renal replacement therapy (dialysis and/or a transplant) one day. But there are things you can do that might delay this and keep your kidneys (and the rest of you) as healthy as possible.

(i) **Keep your blood pressure low.** The kidneys are very sensitive to high blood pressure in diabetic patients. Since kidney disease causes high blood pressure, nearly all diabetics with kidney trouble are on blood pressure drugs. A type of drug known as an **ACE inhibitor**, may provide special protection, but it will not necessarily be suitable for everyone – your doctor will advise you about this. High blood pressure can damage not only the kidneys, but other parts of the body too, so control of blood pressure is vital.

(ii) **Keep your sugar levels under control.** This might help the kidneys to stay healthy for longer. Keeping your blood sugar under control helps prevent problems with your eyes as well.

(iii) **Monitor your blood cholesterol levels.** You can keep your blood cholesterol low by avoiding fatty foods. Many doctors recommend this, particularly if you have diabetes. It may help with any associated heart or circulation problems too.

(iv) **Don't take up smoking, and if you smoke already then stop!** While there may not be direct links with kidney disease, smoking is clearly linked to heart disease and cancer. It is also known to reduce your general level of fitness. So if you have any long term health problems at all, don't smoke. If you need help to quit smoking, ask your GP.

Will my original kidney disease come back and damage a kidney transplant?

It really depends on what caused your kidney failure in the first place. Some diseases do come back and affect the kidney transplant. These include dense deposit disease (DDD), IgA nephropathy, Goodpasture's syndrome, haemolytic uraemic syndrome (HUS) and focal and segmental glomerulosclerosis (FSGS). If you have one of these diseases, the doctors may want to take special precautions, or even delay a transplant until the blood tests that diagnose the disease are negative. Vasculitis and SLE (lupus) recur only rarely. Diabetes, one of the main causes of kidney failure in the UK, does affect the transplanted kidney but it is rare for this to lead to serious damage, particularly if great care is taken with control of diabetes and blood pressure.

In most other patients, the original kidney disease does not come back after a transplant.

Why am I still passing urine if I have kidney failure?

There are two important constituents of urine – water and waste.

The volume of urine you pass shows how much water is being removed from your body but the level of waste in the urine has to be measured in a laboratory. Some patients still pass a lot of urine, but it may contain just a few (or no) waste products. So, the amount of urine passed is not a good guide to the function of your kidneys, it is the 'quality' of the urine that is most important. For example, you could have a glass of wine that looks quite normal, but when you taste it you realise it is poor quality. However, we are not recommending you taste your urine to check the quality!

I am a haemodialysis patient and one of the nurses on the unit has given me a target weight of 80 kg. What is a 'target weight'?

People with healthy kidneys weigh about the same, almost all the time (unless they eat a lot and get fat or are on a diet). This is because their kidneys are able to balance the amount of fluid going into and out of the body. They therefore do not have a 'target weight'.

Kidney patients, on the other hand, are given a target weight (sometimes called a 'dry weight') by the medical team in the renal unit. This is the body's weight when it has exactly the right percentage of water to solids. So, if you have been given a target weight of 80 kg, the medical team has estimated that you should have 48 kg of flesh and 32 kg of water in your body (60% flesh/ 40% water). One litre of water weighs 1 kg and so your body contains 32 litres of fluid.

It is easy to see whether the fluid balance is disturbed. If someone with healthy kidneys drinks one litre of fluid (water, tea, beer etc.) their weight would increase by 1 kg until they pass urine. As you have kidney failure and do not pass much urine, the water will stay in your body (and you will stay 1 kg above your target weight) until the excess fluid is removed by dialysis.

Outcomes

How long can I expect to live after I start dialysis?

The way doctors estimate how long a person will survive with any disease is to look at the percentage chance of living 1, 2, 5 and 10 years after starting treatment. This measurement is used in many diseases, including cancer and heart disease, as well as for dialysis patients. The problem with this way of looking at the figures is that to an individual patient, they don't really mean much. For example, you can see from the table below that after a year of being on dialysis over 80% of patients are still alive. In other words, out of 100 patients who start dialysis, 80 will still be alive a year later and 20 will have died. The figures cannot say which 20 patients will die, or whether they will die because of their kidney failure. They might die from an entirely different cause.

Another important fact is that out of the 20% of dialysis patients who die in the first year, 50% die in the first three months. There could be a number of reasons for this, such as how old the patient is, how sick they were when they started dialysis and what other problems and illnesses they have.

Chances of living	
1 year	80%
2 years	68%
5 years	37%
10 years	21%

It is important to compare the chances of survival of dialysis patients with people who have other serious long-term diseases. For example, the chance of living for five years if you have lung cancer is 27%, and 60% if you have breast cancer. So, it can be seen that the outlook for people with kidney failure is not too good.

Does a transplant make you live any longer than dialysis?

It is difficult to answer this question definitively. This is because it is difficult to compare the results from dialysis and transplant patients. This is because kidney transplant is a major operation and patients need to be pretty fit to go through it in the first place – so often the patients on dialysis are less well to begin with. We are not comparing like with like.

However, some research (using fancy mathematics) has been done in this area. It appears that having a transplant does not make you live longer than you would have done had you stayed on dialysis. This is probably because damage to the heart occurs early in the course of kidney failure, long before you need dialysis or a transplant – indeed long before you meet a kidney doctor. A kidney transplant will certainly improve your quality of life however, if it works well.

Does the cause of my kidney failure make any difference to how long I will live?

Yes – but it is not really the disease that affects how long you will live, it is the complications of the disease. As a general guide, people with polycystic kidney disease have the best chance of survival. This could be because they do not usually have other problems affecting their health such as heart disease or diabetes.

As the table shows, people with high blood pressure or diabetes are not as likely to live for 10 years on dialysis as those with either polycystic kidney disease or glomerulonephritis. This table shows the chances of people surviving 1, 2, 5 and 10 years depending on what has caused their kidney failure.

	1 year	2 years	5 years	10 years
Polycystic kidneys	94	85	70	42
Glomerulonephritis	88	79	58	37
Obstructive nephropathy	82	69	46	21
Unknown cause	76	65	41	19
High blood pressure	77	63	33	14
Diabetes mellitus	79	63	29	11

We are sorry if the disease that caused your kidney failure is not in this table. This is all the data that is currently available.

Do younger people live for longer on dialysis than older people?

Yes, your age does affect how long you are likely to live if you have kidney failure, just as healthy people are more likely to die if they are old. The following table shows the percentage chance of you surviving 1, 2, 5 and 10 years depending on how old you are at the start of dialysis.

	1 year	2 years	5 years	10 years
Younger than 20 years	98	95	88	79
Between 20–44	94	88	71	52
Between 45–64	88	77	44	15
Between 65–74	75	58	21	2
Over 74 years	63	44	10	1

Overall, younger people with kidney failure are likely to live longer than older people – as you might expect. But these figures also show a few unexpected things.

First, look at the chances of the two younger age groups surviving five years (88 and 71%). These are young people by modern standards (the average life expectancy of men and women in the UK is around 80 years). These figures show us that kidney failure is a serious disease that affects their chances of reaching middle age.

Now look at the results for the oldest age group (over 74-year-olds). A large number (44%) of this age group will survive for two years on dialysis. Not many (10%) will live longer than five years. But compare this to their chances of living two or five years if they didn't have kidney failure and you will see that dialysis works well in older people.

Will kidney failure kill me?

This is a simple question but is more complicated than it appears. Probably the most accurate answer is that, while kidney failure isn't often the cause of death, it is likely to shorten your life.

The most common reason that people with kidney failure die is because they have heart disease as well (42%). This is also one of the most common causes of death in the general population of the UK (23%). However, if you have kidney failure, you are much more likely to die of heart problems than if you don't have kidney failure.

This table shows the most common causes of death in people with kidney failure.

	Dialysis	Transplant
Heart disease	42%	30%
Infections	15%	12%
Strokes	12%	12%
Treatment stopped	18%	3%
Cancer	6%	34%
Other	6%	9%

These causes of death are not typical of people in the UK. In most developed countries of the world, most people die of cancer (25%), then heart disease (23%), then strokes (11%). So, although a lot of kidney patients do die from these common diseases, there are other causes of death.

Many people with kidney failure die of infections. In transplant patients, infections are more common because the patient is taking immunosuppressant drugs (see pages 144, 146) to prevent kidney rejection.

Patients with advanced kidney disease may die because they choose to stop dialysis. Some people ask the doctor whether they can do this because they are very unhappy, in a lot of pain or can no longer cope with treatment. Sometimes the doctors and nurses do not think dialysis is giving the patient any quality of life, and might discuss with them whether or not they wish to continue.

Do kidney patients in some geographical areas have a better chance of living longer than patients from others?

Information from the Renal Registry (the national computer system that registers kidney patients) indicates that some areas of the country treat more patients than others; that is, you are more likely to get dialysis or a transplant if you live in a certain region (sometimes referred to as the 'postcode lottery'). This is worrying, because patients with kidney failure will die without dialysis or a transplant.

There are also some areas where patients are more likely to get certain types of treatment than others. For example, EPO (see page 52), APD (see page 96) or home haemodialysis (see page 112). More worryingly, there is a wide range of new patients in different areas – ranging from 55 to 150 new patients per million of the population. It appears that patients from certain regions in the UK are more likely to get dialysis than patients from others.

How many patients are on dialysis in the UK, compared to other European countries?

A useful way of assessing how well (or badly) different countries are meeting their people's need for kidney failure treatment is to use a statistic called the 'take-on rate for dialysis'. This measures the number of new patients per million of the population who start dialysis in any particular year. The latest complete set of European figures is rather old, unfortunately, as it was compiled in 1995. But it does reveal wide variations. One possible explanation for this is that European peoples are not similar – Romanians, for example, do not often develop kidney failure. This seems unlikely. A more plausible explanation is that some countries are better than others at identifying and providing treatment for people who develop kidney failure.

In some countries – notably Norway, Denmark and Sweden – more people with ESRF are likely to be given a transplant without ever starting dialysis.

In 1995, the UK's performance in terms of take-on for dialysis left a lot to be desired. The UK came twelfth, with only half the dialysis take-on rate of the top country, Germany. As in football, we are way behind the Germans. Fortunately for kidney patients, however, the national take-on rate for dialysis is improving. In 1998, the UK took on 96 new dialysis patients per million population, compared to 87 in 1995. These numbers were significantly better than the take-on rate of only 61 in 1993. The provision of dialysis in the UK continues to improve, but the rate of improve-

European Dialysis League, 1995

Positions in this league are determined by the country's take-on rate, ie by the number of new patients per million population who started dialysis in 1995.

1. Germany	163		13. Bulgaria	84
2. Luxembourg	155		14. Netherlands	82
3. Czech Republic	143		15. Norway	80
4. Italy	131		16. Hungary	77
5. Portugal	126		17. Greece	75
6. Spain	121		18. Switzerland	75
7. Belgium	116		19. Ireland	69
8. Austria	115		20. Finland	68
9. France	112		21. Poland	44
10. Sweden	99		22. Iceland	33
11. Denmark	98		23. Romania	26
12. United Kingdom	87			

ment is still far too slow. The most recent figures on treatment for ESRF in the UK and various other countries can be found on the Renal Registry's website – www.renalreg.com.

Are UK patients more likely to have a transplant than patients in the rest of Europe?

Another way of assessing how well different countries are meeting the need for treatment for kidney failure is to compare the number of kidney transplants performed per million population in any one year. Like the take-on rate for dialysis, the rate of kidney transplantation should be similar in all countries. Again, it is easy to see from the 'European Transplant League' table, that this is clearly not the case. Some countries perform many more kidney transplants per million population than others.

The UK has an even worse record in the 'European Transplant League' than in the 'European Dialysis League'. In 1995, the UK came 15th, with 25 transplants per million population. This was lower than in 1994, when the UK was 11th with 30 transplants per million population (even though there were 28 transplants per million population in 1998). The UK clearly has a long way to go

European Transplant League, 1995

Positions in this league are determined by the country's transplant rate, ie by the number of patients per million population who received transplants in 1995.

1.	Norway	56	12.	Belgium	28
2.	Spain	45	13.	Denmark	28
3.	Portugal	38	14.	France	28
4.	Sweden	37	15.	United Kingdom	25
5.	Switzerland	36	16.	Italy	24
6.	Austria	35	17.	Czech Republic	23
7.	Finland	33	18.	Iceland	20
8.	Luxembourg	33	19.	Bulgaria	15
9.	Ireland	32	20.	Greece	14
10.	Germany	30	21.	Poland	10
11.	Netherlands	29	22.	Romania	5

before it matches the performance of the two 'European Transplant League' leaders, Norway and Spain.

One reason why the UK does not come higher in the European Transplant League is that this country has a relatively low death rate from road traffic and industrial accidents. This affects the availability of cadaveric kidneys for transplantation. The situation would be improved if more people registered their willingness to donate their organs for transplantation and discussed their wishes with their next of kin.

Am I more likely to live longer with a living transplant or a cadaveric transplant?

Overall, you have a much better chance of living longer if you have had a living transplant. The following table shows percentage chances of living for 1, 2, 5 and 10 years after a cadaveric transplant, and compares it with a living transplant:

	1 year	2 years	5 years	10 years
Cadaveric	94%	92%	80%	56%
Living	97%	96%	89%	77%

From this table you can see that having a transplant is not without risks; 3% of people who have had a living kidney transplant are dead within a year, and 6% of those who have had a cadaveric kidney transplant will be also be dead within a year.
But, it is important to put these statistics into perspective: 20% of patients die within the first year if they stay on dialysis (see page 34). This is not a fair comparison, as the average age of patients who have a transplant is usually more than 10 years younger than that of patients starting dialysis.

Even though people who have living transplants have a slightly better chance of survival for the first 2 years, at 5 years the picture is very different. A patient with a living transplant has a 10% higher chance of being alive; and at 10 years, a staggering 20% better chance. This may be because living transplants tend to last longer than cadaveric ones. So, after 10 years, people who have had a living transplant are more likely not to be on dialysis and therefore healthier.

3
Treatment of kidney failure

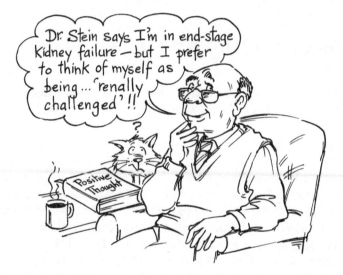

There is currently no cure for kidney failure, although doctors continue to search for one. Some steps can be taken at an early stage to slow down the disease but, for many patients, 'treatment' involves renal replacement therapy (RRT) once their kidneys have failed completely. RRT, which replaces the lost function of the kidneys rather than 'curing' them, takes the form of either dialysis or transplantation. Once you have been diagnosed with kidney failure, you will always have the condition whether you have a transplant or are on dialysis.

There are more than 35,000 patients on dialysis or with a transplant in the UK.

Dialysis is a treatment to remove excess water, waste and salt from the blood and many people are able to carry on with their life while undergoing this treatment. However, if dialysis were stopped, the patient would probably not survive more than a few weeks.

A transplanted kidney performs all the functions of a healthy kidney, so is a more effective treatment than dialysis. But transplants are not without their problems, many of which are addressed in Chapter 6.

Keeping healthy for longer

I am in my late twenties and I have just been diagnosed with kidney failure. What can I do to live longer?

Although people with chronic kidney failure do not live as long as people without any illness, kidney failure is not usually fatal. Only a few people actually die as a direct result of kidney failure. Death occurs either as a result of the disease that caused kidney failure (such as problems caused by diabetes) or from the treatment of kidney failure (dialysis or a transplant).

Heart disease is the main cause of death for kidney patients. Permanent damage to the heart often happens early in kidney failure, before dialysis or a transplant is needed. This damage is probably due to several things, including high blood pressure, anaemia and fluid overload. It is also possible that the wastes that build up in the blood in people with kidney failure have a directly toxic effect on the heart. Neither dialysis nor a transplant can do anything to repair an already damaged heart.

If you are a young patient with kidney failure, it is important you look after yourself properly. Eat a diet that is fresh, healthy and low in salt. Make sure you are not anaemic (see Chapter 2), and your blood pressure is kept normal or low by taking blood pressure tablets (see page 29). It is also important that you are well dialysed (see Chapter 5) and never have fluid overload (see page 56). Limiting the amount you drink might help you to avoid fluid overload. Don't smoke and keep your heart and muscles strong and healthy by taking regular exercise.

The best long term form of treatment is a transplant from a living donor (see Chapter 5). If you can arrange to have this transplant before you need dialysis, and if the transplant works well, you will have a good chance of living for a long time.

The doctor tells me that my kidneys have about 20% function left. I feel terrible and there are all sorts of things I can't eat or do. When I go onto dialysis, will I be able to have a normal life again the rest of the time?

Certainly, you should feel better when you start dialysis, but you do need to be aware that you still have a part to play in helping yourself to feel as well as possible. Dialysis removes excess water and certain wastes from the body, but the function of a healthy kidney is more complex than this. It also has an important role in carefully controlling the levels of many substances in the blood, and often in conserving them where necessary. So, if your kidneys fail, you are likely to suffer from a variety of problems. Your blood pressure may go up, and the level of fats in your blood will also rise. Your haemoglobin (the oxygen carrying pigment in the red cells of your blood) may go down and you will become anaemic. Your bones may ache because of disturbances in the amount of calcium and phosphate in them. Continuing to eat a healthy diet, low in saturated fats and salt, is important. Avoid processed foods, ready meals and fast foods, all of which may have hidden high levels of salt and fat content. You will also need to be very careful about how much fluid you drink.

You may be given tablets to control your blood pressure but, like dialysis, you will get most benefit from these if you do as much as you can for your own health too. Anaemia is usually treated by injections of erythropoietin (EPO, see page 52).

I have heard that salt is bad for the kidneys – but I never use it on my food. So how can this be true, and even if it were, what could I do about it?

If you have kidney disease, you are advised to avoid salt for two main reasons. Firstly, many people with kidney disease suffer from high blood pressure which if left untreated can damage your heart and circulatory system. Secondly, it is very important that you restrict your fluid intake in order to avoid fluid overload (see page 56). Eating salty food will inevitably make you more thirsty so it will be harder to control how much fluid you drink.

A major problem for anyone seeking to reduce how much salt they eat is that many foods, particularly fast foods, 'junk' foods and ready-prepared foods, contain a lot of 'hidden' salt. You should try to avoid these wherever possible. If you do buy some occasionally, check the ingredient labels carefully.

Do I need a special diet because I have kidney failure?

Diet is important in the treatment of renal failure as many of the waste products that build up in the blood come from the food that you eat. You may be advised to modify your diet to help control sodium, potassium, phosphate, protein and fluid. Cutting down on salt is important (see above).

Many people with renal failure are referred to a dietitian to discuss their diet. Dietitians are experts in advising people on how to balance their diets to suit their medical condition. Although your dietitian may specialise in diets for people with renal failure, he or she will consider any other problems you may have, such as diabetes or high blood cholesterol levels.

Are there any diets that are dangerous for people with kidney failure?

You should always check with your dietitian before taking any form of vitamin or mineral supplements or any health food product. Any diet which causes an imbalance of nutrients can be a problem. Diets which restrict or encourage a large number of particular foods or types of food can be especially dangerous if you have kidney failure. Examples include the 'Grapefruit diet', 'Very Low Calorie diets,' 'Macrobiotic diet' and 'body-building diets.' Your dietitian will give you more detailed advice.

My brother has advanced kidney failure and will soon be on dialysis. Should he go on a low protein diet? Could it do him any harm?

In the past 'low protein diets' were used to treat kidney failure, especially before dialysis was readily available. There are some people who believe that 'low protein diets' may delay the need for dialysis but scientific studies designed to show this were limited and have been superseded by a large study in the USA showing low protein diets to be of no benefit. Furthermore, people with kidney failure are often unable to eat enough to meet their nutritional needs and lose weight or become malnourished anyway. A 'low protein diet' may make this worse, and most doctors no longer agree with its use.

My mum is on peritoneal dialysis and is becoming weak. She has barely any appetite and has a very low protein level in her blood. How can we get back her appetite and her strength?

There are many reasons why people may lose their appetite on peritoneal dialysis (PD). Some people have poor appetites because they feel full very quickly. They often cannot finish a meal because of the pressure of the dialysis fluid on the stomach. The answer is to try small meals and snacks often throughout the day (every two hours for example). It may help to avoid bulky or filling foods such as too much fruit/vegetables or fizzy drinks and avoid drinking with meals. The dietitian may be able to suggest ways in which meals can be fortified, or recommend nutritional supplements. It might be worth talking to the dialysis nurse to see whether your mother is receiving enough dialysis, as loss of appetite can be associated with poor dialysis.

I'm on HD and losing body weight. I have very little appetite but am anxious I'm not keeping to my low potassium diet. What can I do?

Firstly you should let your dietitian know, so that he or she can advise you on fortifying your food or taking appropriate supplements. The main issue here is that you are not taking in enough energy and protein. It is unlikely that you will be getting too much potassium through the small amount of food that you are eating. If this potassium is coming from fruit and vegetables, these are also likely to fill you up without providing much energy or protein. You should swap the fruit and vegetables for more energy/protein rich foods such as sandwiches, bread and butter or biscuits. Try to eat small regular meals and snacks. You could also try including more fatty foods in your diet to give you more energy while your appetite is poor.

My doctor is always telling me that that my phosphate level is high. Why is this a problem and what can I do about it?

High levels of phosphate in the blood can cause unpleasant itching and eventually can cause your bones to become weak and brittle (renal bone disease, see pages 58–61). Certain foods (for example, dairy produce, offal and eggs) contain a large amount of phosphate. By limiting the amount of these foods in your diet you can help to control your blood phosphate level. Another way in which you can control your phosphate level is to ensure that you are taking your phosphate binding tablets correctly (Calcichew, Titralac, Phosex). These need to be taken just before your meal.

Why do I need vitamin D tablets? Doesn't the body get all the vitamin D it needs from my ordinary diet?

Normally this is true, but if you have kidney failure the body is unable to make use of the vitamin D you eat. This means you will need to take an active form of the vitamin (such as Alfacalcidol) as a supplement.

Symptoms and what to do about them

What are the symptoms of kidney failure?

In the early stages of kidney failure there are often no symptoms. Later on, some or all of the following may be experienced:

- itching
- tiredness and weakness
- loss of appetite
- poor concentration
- restless legs
- leg cramps
- swollen ankles
- shortness of breath
- poor sleeping
- poor sex drive
- feeling cold
- alteration in taste.

My husband has bad kidney failure, and is approaching the need for dialysis. One of the symptoms he is experiencing is altered taste. To him even the nicest food tastes awful. He can only drink water as everything else (tea, coffee etc.) is unpalatable. How can he be helped?

It is common for patients with kidney failure to experience altered taste. It is caused by the build-up of toxins in the blood. This unpleasant symptom may well disappear when he starts to have treatment and the levels of toxins in the body are reduced.

Even though it isn't pleasant, it is important that he continues to eat a healthy diet while waiting to start dialysis.

I have polycystic disease and sometimes I pass red urine. Should I be worried?

Sometimes, the cysts on your kidneys can burst or get infected and this can make your urine turn red because there is blood in it. However, blood in the urine can have other causes. So it is always important to tell the doctors in the renal unit if you notice your urine has changed colour.

Infection can be diagnosed by testing a sample of your urine. You may be given antibiotics and can take painkillers if necessary.

Other complications of polycystic disease include cysts in your liver, high blood pressure and an increased chance of having a stroke.

My doctor says I have glomerulonephritis, but I feel very well and don't have any pain. Has the doctor made a mistake?

Whatever the cause of kidney failure, many patients have no symptoms in the early stages and most feel completely well. The only signs of damage to the kidneys may be small amounts of blood or protein, detectable only by special tests, in the urine. It is rare for inflamed kidneys to cause pain.

Why do I itch so much? Can anything be done about it?

Itching is one of the most common problems experienced by patients with kidney failure, and unfortunately one of the hardest to treat. Many patients find it extremely distressing, particularly at night.

No one knows exactly what causes itching, but some doctors believe it is related to high phosphate levels in the blood. Reducing phosphate in the diet and taking calcium carbonate may improve itching in some patients.

The doctor may be able to prescribe anti-itching drugs such as Piriton, but this is not effective for all patients. Some people find applying moisturising cream or calamine lotion helps to soothe the itchiness.

If none of these measures work, the doctor may suggest an increase in dialysis.

My husband is on peritoneal dialysis. He sleeps very little and is very restless at night. This disturbs my sleep too, and I am getting tired. Would sleeping pills help?

The first question to ask is why your husband is so restless. It may be that some of the symptoms of kidney failure such as itching, restless legs or cramps cause his poor sleep. If this is the case you should discuss it with his renal doctor. The symptoms may be due to the fact that he isn't getting enough dialysis and he might need more. The doctor may be able to prescribe something to help, such as a short course of Clonazepam or similar tablets. Although not a long-term solution (and probably not a good idea for you!) tablets may help him re-establish a normal sleeping pattern.

You certainly need your sleep, to have the energy to cope and to help with his care. Some couples decide to have separate beds, or even separate rooms, due to this problem. However, if the problem can be solved in any other way, it is probably better for the relationship.

Will kidney failure affect my mouth? What can I do about it?

It can do. Most patients experience a dry mouth. Other effects include a metallic taste, bad breath, inflamed gums, frequent mouth ulcers and loose teeth. As there is an increase in tooth decay, it is important to brush teeth more regularly, and for longer – preferably with an electric toothbrush, twice a day. It is also a good idea to see a dental hygienist at least twice a year, as you may need your teeth polished. This does not hurt!

Would it be helpful to use a mouthwash?

Routine use of a mouthwash is not recommended. Most mouthwashes contain acid and ethanol (a type of alcohol). These ingredients alter the balance of bacteria (bugs) in the mouth and are not helpful. In addition, ethanol tends to dry out the mouth, exacerbating a common problem in kidney patients.

I have been feeling very tired and breathless and my doctor says I am anaemic. What does this mean?

Blood is made up of two parts: a liquid part and a more solid part. The liquid part is called plasma. It accounts for about 60% of the blood's volume, and is mainly water. The amount of water in the plasma is increased in fluid overload and decreased in dehydration.

The other 40% of the blood is made up of blood cells, which are so tiny they can only be seen through a microscope. There are various different types of cells: red cells (which carry oxygen around the body), white cells (which fight infection) and platelets (involved in blood clotting). Most of the blood cells are red cells. These give the blood its red colour. Each one looks rather like a tiny doughnut. Red cells are smaller than white cells, and larger than platelets. You have about 5 million red cells in one drop of blood. Anaemia is due to a shortage of haemoglobin (or Hb, the oxygen-carrying substance in the red blood cells) and is probably the most important complication of kidney failure. It is the main reason why people on dialysis feel weak and tired. In fact, many of the symptoms of kidney failure are not caused by kidney failure but are actually due to anaemia.

The main symptoms of anaemia are breathlessness, tiredness, pale skin, poor appetite, irritability and low sex drive.

I have been diagnosed with kidney failure and I have started dialysis. I have now been told that I am anaemic. What have my kidneys got to do with my blood?

The main reason you have developed anaemia is simple. One of the extra jobs the kidneys do is to help make red blood cells in the bone marrow. To do this, your kidneys make a substance called **erythropoietin** (abbreviated to **EPO**). This is a natural substance, but it can now be artificially produced and given to people who don't produce enough of their own.

EPO travels around your body in the blood from the kidneys to the bone marrow, where it constantly reminds your bone marrow to keep producing red cells. Because you have kidney failure, your kidneys may make less EPO than normal. So the bone marrow 'goes to sleep' and makes fewer red cells. As a result, anaemia develops, and you may become weak and tired.

There are other reasons why kidney patients become anaemic. For example, red blood cells do not live as long as normal (120 days) in people with kidney failure, and so must be replaced more rapidly. Also, blood may be lost during haemodialysis, or through frequent blood tests.

Do I have to wait until I get bone pain before renal bone disease can be diagnosed?

Renal bone disease does not necessarily cause pain.

Testing levels of calcium and phosphate in your blood can tell us what is happening in the bones at the time of the test. However, these levels provide little information about the future.

The best guide to the progress and severity of renal bone disease is the amount of parathyroid hormone (PTH) in your blood. PTH tells us much more about the long term health of your bones. Changes in blood PTH can tell us about what will happen to your bones in the future – the lower the PTH, the better. However, the levels of PTH, calcium and phosphate in your blood have no bearing on the severity of pain you may get with renal bone disease. Some patients with fairly normal levels may have severe pain, while others with abnormal levels may have no pain at all.

Renal bone disease begins very early in kidney failure. So it is a good idea for your doctor to measure your blood PTH even before dialysis is necessary. Once dialysis has started, most doctors will measure your blood PTH every six months or so. A high level indicates a problem with the bones. Doctors will then start a range of treatments to help prevent any worsening of the problem. Even very high PTH levels can usually be lowered with the right tablets.

If your renal bone disease does cause you pain, ask your doctor if you can be referred to a specialist pain clinic.

Will all the problems I have been getting with my blood phosphate and calcium levels go away when I have a transplant?

If you receive a transplant and the new kidney works well, the blood levels of calcium, phosphate, vitamin D and PTH will usually return to normal, or near normal. Renal bone disease then improves, although it never goes away completely.

If your transplanted kidney never functions properly, or if it starts to fail after working well, renal bone disease will become a problem again. It is important to pay attention to the calcium, phosphate and PTH levels even after your transplant.

Can anything be done to treat my anaemia and make me feel better?

The usual treatment for anaemia is with a substance called **erythropoietin (EPO)**, which is given as an injection one to three times per week. This is a naturally occurring substance produced by the bone marrow when it is stimulated by a kidney in good working order. Fortunately, EPO can now be made synthetically and given to those people who are unable to produce enough of their own.

Dialysis patients who are not being treated with EPO may have an Hb of only 6–8 grams per decilitre of blood (g/dl), which is very low. The aim of EPO treatment is to increase the Hb level to 10–12 grams per decilitre.

In the past the only way to improve the haemoglobin was by giving the patient blood transfusions. One problem with these is that they can only raise the haemoglobin for a few weeks. Another problem is that every time a patient has a blood transfusion they build up substances called **antibodies** in the blood to protect themselves from the 'foreign' cells in the transfused blood. These antibodies stay in the body for many years and if the patient has a transplant they can attack the new kidney, so that it is rejected.

These days there is no reason for patients to have blood

transfusions to cure their anaemia if EPO is given as soon as anaemia is discovered.

For EPO to work well, however, the body must have sufficient stores of iron. The best guide to how much iron there is in the body is the blood test to measure the level of serum ferritin. The more iron there is in the body, the higher the level of ferritin in the blood. If EPO is to work, it is important that the ferritin level is at least 200 mg/l (milligrams per litre of blood). To keep the ferritin above this level, many patients on EPO have to take iron tablets, or to have regular iron injections. (The injections do hurt a little, by the way.) Some renal units now give iron injections to all patients with kidney failure, whether they are on EPO or not.

I have been taking EPO three times a week for five months but my Hb is still only 7.8 g/dl. The doctors aren't doing anything – what should I do?

Most people should respond to regular treatment with EPO, however, it sometimes takes a few months to start working properly. When it does start working, EPO improves all the symptoms of anaemia.

However, it may not work if you have another problem such as:

- **Infection** especially repeated peritonitis (in PD patients), and dialysis catheter infections (in haemodialysis patients).
- **Under-dialysis** may also prevent EPO from working well (see page 120).
- **Severe renal bone disease** (see page 51).
- **Iron deficiency** (which can be diagnosed by a blood test to measure ferritin, see page 79) is the most common reason for EPO not to work. Iron deficiency can sometimes be treated with iron tablets (usually a type called ferrous sulphate), or by regular iron injections. Iron tablets can make you constipated and turn your stools black. Black stools are nothing to worry about, but you should ask your doctor's advice on avoiding constipation.
- **Malignancy (cancer)** – especially myeloma.

If EPO stops working for whatever reason, or if you stop taking it, your Hb will return to the 'normal' low level in people with kidney failure (usually 6–8 g/dl). The symptoms of anaemia will then return.

I have not started dialysis yet. Do I need to take EPO?

Anaemia begins long before kidney patients need to start dialysis. Therefore some doctors now give EPO injections before dialysis is needed. You can find out if you need EPO by asking the doctors or nurses in clinic if you are anaemic. If your Hb is below 10 g/dl you should be given EPO.

EPO may also be given if a transplant is failing, as anaemia often returns at this time.

My blood pressure has risen since I started taking EPO. Is this a side effect?

Yes, the only common side effect of EPO is worsening of high blood pressure. This appears to be more likely in people who have had severe high blood pressure in the past, or in people who are on more than one type of blood pressure tablet.

If the blood pressure does increase, you may need to take more blood pressure tablets. You should never stop taking your EPO injections unless you have been told to by your EPO nurse or kidney doctor.

A combination of EPO and high blood pressure can sometimes cause epileptic fits, but this problem can usually be prevented by treating the high blood pressure.

I have been on haemodialysis for over two years. Will I ever be able to stop EPO injections?

Some people, after many years on dialysis, start making their own EPO again. This is rare, but if it does happen, the haemoglobin starts to rise for no apparent reason and the person may be able to stop EPO injections. Most people who have a successful transplant can stop taking EPO, as the new kidney will start to make it.

Since I started taking EPO, I've started getting erections again. It's great and my girlfriend's 'over the moon'. If I double the dose, will that give me more erections?

Curing anaemia (raising the Hb) often has an effect on sex drive, enabling men to have erections if they have had this difficulty since getting kidney failure. However, increasing the dose of EPO (even if it does raise the Hb further), will not affect the number of erections you have – sorry!

It is never safe to alter the dose of EPO without consulting your doctor or EPO nurse. Furthermore, EPO is a very expensive drug (£2,000–4,000 per year for each patient) and so another reason for not increasing the dose, if a low dose is effective for you, is to enable more patients to be given it.

I don't mind having to take EPO, but would rather not if I didn't have to. Will I still need it if I have a transplant?

After you have a kidney transplant and it works, your new kidney will start making EPO and the problem of anaemia usually goes away. If this happens you will no longer need EPO injections. However, if your transplant kidney ever fails, anaemia will usually return, and EPO injections may be needed again.

I'm always being told off by the doctors and nurses in the renal unit because I drink too much. But I'm thirsty all the time.

Some doctors and nurses may appear to be scolding, but this is not their intention. It is often easier and quicker for medical staff to instruct patients to 'do things' rather than explain the reasons behind these instructions. People with kidney failure are less able to remove water from the body because they only pass a little, if any, urine. There are good reasons, therefore, for advising you to restrict the amount of fluid you drink.

There are other ways in which we can get rid of water – through sweating, breath and faeces. On a normal day, an average person will lose about 500 millilitres of fluid from the body in this way. So, most people who pass no urine at all could drink 500 millilitres of liquid a day without it building up. As a general rule therefore it is acceptable for patients to drink 500 millilitres of fluid every day, plus a further amount equal to the volume of urine passed the previous day. In this way, only fluid that has been lost is replaced so there is no danger of excess fluid building up in the body.

Many patients complain of excessive thirst and this can be a problem. It is particularly difficult to stop doing something (drinking) when it is a lifelong habit, particularly if you are being told not to do it! Restricting fluid intake will never be easy, but it is extremely important if you have kidney failure.

There are a number of different tactics for overcoming thirst. These include chewing gum, cutting down on salt, sucking ice-cubes or slices of lemon. It is also possible to fool yourself into thinking you are not restricting your fluid intake by drinking the same number of drinks each day but using a smaller cup.

I am told my swollen ankles are caused by fluid overload. This doesn't bother me so why is it such a problem?

Fluid overload occurs when there is too much fluid in the body (the balance between flesh and fluid is wrong) and it can be very dangerous. It is usually caused by drinking too much fluid or (if you are on dialysis) by not having efficient dialysis.

If you are fluid overloaded you may have:

  (i) swelling, particularly in the ankles, hands and around the eyes;

 (ii) breathlessness;

(iii) a sudden increase in weight;

(iv) high blood pressure (you cannot tell if you have high blood pressure unless it is measured with a blood pressure machine).

If your body becomes badly fluid overloaded or fluid overloaded on a regular basis, a lot of damage can be done. In extreme cases the excess fluid will remain in the lungs making it difficult for you to breathe. Too much fluid in the circulation causes your blood pressure to rise and this can put a strain on your heart. Over a long period this will enlarge the heart and make the heart muscles weak, which can be fatal.

Two things can be done to rectify fluid overload. The first is to stop drinking. Any more liquid taken in will make the situation worse. The second is to remove the excess fluid from the body. This can be done in two ways. One of these is with dialysis, if you are on it:

- **Haemodialysis** removes fluid efficiently and the machine can be set up so that it accurately removes just the right amount of fluid over a specified time.
- **Peritoneal dialysis (PD)** is also good at getting rid of excess fluid. This is usually done by using stronger bags of PD solution (see page 105).

The other way applies only if the kidneys are still able to make urine (either before you have started dialysis or if you have a transplant that is failing), and involves taking 'water' tablets or **diuretics** (eg Frusemide).

I'm on haemodialysis and have terrible trouble with ankle swelling. I can't fit into my shoes any more. Can you tell me how to make it better?

Ankle swelling is one of the main symptoms of fluid overload – excess fluid has built up in and under the skin. The best way to reduce the swelling is to drink less and remove the fluid by having more dialysis (see above). You should be aware that some foods, such as sauces, soups or custards, themselves contain a lot of water. Also, cutting down on your salt intake will make you feel less thirsty.

However, it may be difficult to get rid of the swelling in some patients, particularly if they have low levels of **albumin** in the blood. Albumin is a form of protein that helps to move fluid out of the tissues and into the bloodstream so that it can be removed by dialysis. The normal level of albumin in the blood is between 35 and 50 grams per litre. It is quite difficult to raise your albumin levels but you could try eating more protein-rich foods such as eggs, meat and fish.

I feel dizzy and weak. I have been told I am dehydrated. What does this mean?

Dehydration is the opposite of fluid overload and is usually caused by losing too much fluid. In kidney patients who do not pass much urine, this is rare. But it can happen if the patient has lost fluid in some other way, for example through vomiting and diarrhoea.

If you have dehydration you may experience dizziness (caused by low blood pressure), dry skin and weight loss.

The best treatment for dehydration is to replace the lost fluid by drinking more. In very severe cases this is not possible and it may be necessary to have fluid intravenously in hospital via a drip.

If you are on diuretics ('water tablets'), these may need to be reduced for a while. If you are on dialysis, the nurses should take off less fluid.

I am often kept awake at night with really bad leg cramps. What causes them and how can I stop them?

Many patients experience this unpleasant symptom, which is thought to be caused by an imbalance of sodium (salt) and water in the body. It may be helpful to take a tablet called Quinine, which can alleviate cramp.

Our main concern at the moment is that my husband, a haemodialysis patient, is suffering very badly with aching legs and hips. They ache all the time when he's sitting, standing or walking. Why is this happening?

The kidneys are responsible for maintaining strong and healthy bones. Healthy kidneys help with the absorption of calcium from food that we eat, and it is calcium that helps to keep the bones strong. Some patients who have had kidney failure for a long time, and have not been able to maintain the correct balance of calcium in their body, may develop renal bone disease (see below). This may be the cause of your husband's pain.

There are other reasons why patients get pain in the bones, including a condition known as dialysis amyloid. Osteoarthritis is also a common cause of pain in older people – whether or not they have kidney failure. If correction of your husband's renal bone disease does not relieve his pain, his doctor should look for these and other diseases.

I have a lot of pain in my back and my doctor told me this is because I have renal bone disease. How can my kidneys have anything to do with the health of my bones?

Most people with kidney failure have some degree of renal bone disease. This is because one of the 'extra' functions of the kidneys is to help make the bones strong and healthy. For the bones to be strong, the kidneys must be able to maintain a healthy balance of various substances – including calcium, phosphate and vitamin D – in the body. Kidney failure results in abnormal levels of these substances, thus leading to renal bone disease which can cause back pain.

What causes renal bone disease?

Although there are many causes of renal bone disease, three main factors are involved:

(i) **High phosphate levels in the blood**
Phosphate is a mineral that strengthens the bones. Foods that contain phosphate include protein rich substances such as dairy products, nuts and meat, and it may be better to cut down on the amount of these you eat if you have a phosphate problem. But don't do this unless your doctor tells you to.

Like calcium, phosphate is stored in the body in the bones and is also present in the blood. The kidneys normally help to keep the right amount in the blood – not too much, not too little. In people with kidney failure, phosphate builds up in the blood.

The normal level of phosphate in the blood is 0.8 to 1.4

mmol/l. In kidney patients, it is common for the blood phosphate level to be high, rising to more than 2.0 mmol/l. Unfortunately, it is quite difficult to keep phosphate levels normal. High phosphate levels are also thought to cause itching.

(ii) **Low calcium levels in the blood**

Calcium is another mineral that strengthens the bones. It is obtained from some foods, especially dairy products, eggs and green vegetables. Like phosphate, calcium is stored in the bones. There is also some calcium in the blood. The kidneys normally help to keep calcium in the bones. In people with kidney failure, calcium drains out of the bones and is lost from the body. This leads to a fall in the level of calcium in the blood.

The normal blood calcium level is between 2.2 and 2.6 mmol/l (millimoles per litre of blood). In kidney patients, the level of calcium in the blood may fall below 2.0 mmol/l. Treatment can keep the calcium level up quite easily.

(iii) **Low vitamin D levels in the blood**

Vitamin D is needed in the body so that calcium from the diet can be absorbed into the body and used to strengthen the bones. Vitamin D is found in some foods, especially margarine and butter. However, some of our vitamin D is made by the skin (a process that only occurs if the skin is exposed to sunlight). The kidneys are responsible for transforming vitamin D into a form that is usable by the body.

Blood levels of this useable form are not routinely measured because the blood test is expensive and difficult to do. If they were measured, they would be low.

It is quite easy to provide additional vitamin D as tablets or injections, though not all kidney patients need it. Often, it will be enough just to control the levels of calcium and phosphate.

Doctors do not know which of the three main causes of renal bone disease comes first. Nor do they know what leads to what.

But they do know that, although any one of these causes can lead to problems, a combination of the three is usually present in people with kidney failure. More importantly, each of the causes tends to have a 'knock-on' effect, worsening the other two abnormalities. For example, a high phosphate level tends to lower the calcium level, and vice versa. It is important, therefore, to treat all three causes.

I am on dialysis and I have pain in my joints, knees and elbows. I have been told this is due to renal bone disease. Is there anything that can be done to treat it and get rid of the pain?

Each of the three main causes of renal bone disease should be treated, as described below. However, effective treatment is difficult and you may continue to suffer symptoms.

(i) **Lowering your high phosphate levels**
Dialysis removes some phosphate from the blood, but does not do this very efficiently. Most patients may, therefore, need further treatment to control their phosphate levels. The best way of doing this is by taking tablets called 'phosphate binders'. Calcium carbonate is a phosphate binder, as are Renagel and aluminium hydroxide (though the latter is not often used these days). To be effective, any type of phosphate binder needs to be taken just before food, and not together with iron tablets.

If the combination of dialysis and phosphate-binding tablets fails to control your phosphate levels, it may be necessary for you to have more dialysis, or to eat less high-phosphate foods, or both.

Even with treatment, your blood phosphate rarely returns to the normal level of 0.8 to 1.4 mmol/l. So, the target level is less than 1.8 mmol/l.

(ii) **Raising your low calcium levels**
Your body gets some extra calcium from your dialysis fluid. This happens because there is more calcium in the

dialysis fluid than in the blood. Calcium passes from the stronger solution (the dialysis fluid) into the patient's blood (the weaker solution) by a process called **diffusion**. For many kidney patients, extra calcium from dialysis is not enough. They need to take additional calcium carbonate in the form of a preparation called Calcichew. This comes in large tablets that don't taste pleasant, but they may need to be taken daily. Treatment is most successful when blood calcium levels are about 2.5 to 2.6 mmol/l.

(iii) **Raising your low vitamin D levels**

In a few patients, renal bone disease continues to be a problem even when the blood calcium and phosphate levels are brought under control. You may then need treatment with a supplement of 'activated' vitamin D (the usable form). The most common are Alfacalcidol and Calcitrol. Vitamin D treatment works in two ways: it provides the vitamin D that is lacking, and it increases blood calcium levels (see above). If you are on PD, you may receive vitamin D in the form of a tablet. If you are a haemodialysis patient, you may receive it either as a tablet, or as an injection given during dialysis.

I have been asked to take a high dose of calcitriol but it stops me sleeping at night. Why?

There is no reason for your calcitriol to stop you sleeping. Your sleepless nights are more likely to be a symptom of kidney failure itself. But you should tell your doctor about any symptoms you have, as they may be linked to tablets – ie, you may be the world's first case of that problem being caused by a particular tablet.

Patients often link bad things to tablets – understandable as no-one likes taking them and problems are common in kidney failure. However, tablets are not often the cause of problems, though they are easy to blame.

My doctor has told me my calcium and phosphate blood levels are wrong despite taking my Calcichew and Alfacalcidol religiously. He is now telling me I need an operation to remove my parathyroid glands. How are these things connected?

Parathyroid hormone (PTH) is a substance produced by four tiny glands called the parathyroid glands. These glands are situated in the front of the neck. When someone has kidney failure, the parathyroid glands become over-active and produce too much PTH. Raised PTH levels can aggravate renal bone disease. In most patients, correcting the blood levels of calcium, phosphate and vitamin D is enough to control renal bone disease, and to cause PTH levels to fall.

If your doctor has suggested removing your parathyroid glands (a parathyroidectomy), it appears the normal treatment plan has not been enough, and your blood PTH levels have continued to rise.

This may have caused your blood calcium to rise higher than normal (it is usually low in patients with kidney failure). At this stage, your blood phosphate is also likely to be very high. This combination of an extremely high PTH, a high calcium and a very high phosphate level cannot be treated by dialysis and tablets alone. It is necessary to carry out an operation to remove the parathyroid glands.

Without an operation, the blood vessels can become 'furred up' with calcium, which can be dangerous – especially if this applies to the blood vessels around the heart. Calcium may also be deposited in the eyes (making them red and itchy) or in the skin (which can cause parts of the skin to go black and die). A parathyroidectomy is usually a very effective operation. It returns blood calcium levels to normal, and can prevent these complications.

The operation takes 1–2 hours, and requires a hospital stay of 5–7 days. For a few weeks after surgery, you will need frequent blood calcium checks. This is because blood calcium levels can fall very low after the operation. Many patients need to take high doses of calcium carbonate and/or vitamin D after a parathyroidectomy. These can usually be stopped later.

My son has been diagnosed with vasculitis. The doctors have started him on cyclophosphamide. They said his hair may fall out. Will it grow back?

Cyclophosphamide belongs to a group of drugs called immuno-suppressants. As the name suggests, the function of these drugs is to dampen down the immune system, the body's natural defence system. It is used to try to improve kidney function and to dampen down vasculitis, stopping it from causing any further damage to the body. It is often given in high doses to start with, followed by a smaller daily dose.

Like all medicines, cyclophosphamide can cause side effects. With higher doses feeling sick is common. This can be reduced with anti-sickness tablets.

The number of 'white blood cells' in the blood may fall. Your son's blood will be checked regularly to make sure this doesn't occur. Cyclophosphamide can cause inflammation of the bladder, causing blood in the urine. So with higher doses a tablet called Mesna can be given to protect the bladder.

Cyclophosphamide can make people less fertile, and can even result in some never being able to have children. So, if your son is old enough, he should ask the doctors to freeze a sample of his sperm (women can have their eggs or part of their ovaries frozen too) for use in the future. The drug itself is harmful to unborn babies, so contraception should be used while the drug is being taken and for three months afterwards.

Hair loss can occur during treatment. It is more likely with higher doses of cyclophosphamide. After the treatment is finished, his hair will grow back. With lower doses it often comes back before the end of treatment.

I have been told I am two years away from dialysis. I get a lot of headaches. Is it alright to take aspirin?

Aspirin belongs to a group of drugs called **non-steroidal anti-inflammatory drugs** (or **NSAIDs**), which are used for arthritis, headaches, coughs and colds, and period pain. All the drugs from this group should be avoided, because they can also cause the kidneys to fail completely and cause you to need dialysis earlier than expected. (The same would also be true if you had a failing transplant by the way.) There are many types of NSAID. Common ones are "Anadin" (aspirin), "Brufen" or "Nurofen" (ibuprofen) and "Voltarol" (diclofenac). Most of these are available over the counter at your chemist. They should not be used without discussing the risks and benefits with your doctor.

If you get headaches, you could take paracetamol instead.

I have renal artery stenosis, and my kidney function is poor at about 20%. I am not on dialysis yet. I have been put on loads of drugs. I sometimes forget to take them but nothing happens. Is there any need for them and are there any drugs to avoid?

You may have been put on tablets to prevent blood clots, blood pressure tablets and tablets to reduce the cholesterol level in the blood. These may all help your general health. You are right that nothing will happen if you miss the occasional tablet. They are drugs that are designed to prevent things happening in the long term, rather than straightaway.

However, there is a group of drugs which may cause particular complications in people with renal artery stenosis, and which should be avoided if possible. These drugs are used to treat high blood pressure or heart failure. There are two types of these:

(i) **ACE inhibitors** which have names ending in '-pril' (examples are capto**pril,** also called Capoten, lisino**pril,** also called Zestril, enala**pril**, rami**pril** and fosino**pril**).
(ii) **A2 antagonists,** which have names ending '-sartan' (examples include lo**sartan**, irbe**sartan** and cande**sartan**).

Both groups should be avoided because they can cause complete kidney failure if you have renal artery stenosis, making dialysis necessary earlier than expected. Occasionally your doctor will advise it is safe to stay on these drugs if you are already on them.

You might well ask 'why then should they be given?' They are effective in the treatment of high blood pressure and heart failure. Both these conditions are very common, but only a few people who have them will also have renal artery stenosis, which is very rare.

Treatment of end stage renal failure

I am 32 years old with 'early kidney failure'. I've been told it may get worse one day. I'm not sure if I believe that, I feel fine now. In fact, I often miss appointments and nothing happens. This might seem a stupid question, but why should kidney failure be treated?

It is true that people in early kidney failure do not always have symptoms and, like you, they may feel fine. However, the progress of the disease needs to be monitored, as your kidneys are likely to fail completely one day. This is called ESRF. If you are not then treated by dialysis or a transplant, you will develop severe kidney failure symptoms (see page 47) and, after only a few weeks, you will die.

Given the terrible result if no treatment is given, it may seem stupid to ask: 'Why should kidney failure be treated?' The answer seems obvious – 'to keep you alive'. To a certain extent this is true. Once people (and you) have ESRF, they will die without treatment.

So, yes, the main purpose of the treatment of ESRF is to keep you alive. But there is little point in keeping you alive if your quality of life is so poor that you don't want to be alive.

There are, in fact, several reasons why treatment is given to patients with kidney failure (and will be offered to you, even if you miss appointments). It will not only prolong your life, but will also make you feel better and return you to a good quality of life. To achieve this, the two main functions of the kidneys – removing toxins (waste products, see pages 4–5) and maintaining the body's fluid balance (see page 4) – have to be performed for you. Dialysis and transplantation can perform both these vital functions.

When I develop ESRF, how will it be treated?

ESRF can be treated by dialysis or by a kidney transplant. It is usual for a patient to undergo a period of dialysis before transplantation is considered. Dialysis and transplantation provide alternative ways of taking over the work of the patient's failed kidneys.

- **Dialysis**
  In this treatment, some of the work of the kidneys is performed by artificial means. There are two main types of dialysis: peritoneal dialysis (PD) and haemodialysis. Both of these are described in detail in Chapter 4. Both PD and haemodialysis provide about 5% of the function of two normal kidneys.

- **Transplantation**
  This treatment involves the removal of a normal kidney from one person (the donor), and its insertion into a patient with kidney failure (the recipient). Transplantation is done by a surgeon during a transplant operation. A 'good' transplant provides about 50% of the function of two normal kidneys. Transplantation is described in detail in Chapter 5.

My doctor says I will have to start dialysis very soon as my creatinine level is very high at 776 micromoles per litre. How do the doctors know when to start dialysis?

Dialysis is usually started either when you have severe symptoms of kidney failure (going off your food is one of them) which affect normal daily life, or when the level of toxins (and/or water) in the body is so high that it becomes life-threatening. A blood creatinine level of 800 micromoles per litre is generally taken to indicate this point, and is the onset of ESRF. If it is over 1000, this is extremely serious and dialysis may need to be started urgently. Most doctors now usually try to start patients on dialysis when their blood creatinine level is about 600 micromoles per litre (ie just before the onset of ESRF). However, decisions affecting patients should always be made on an individual basis – usually taking into account both your creatinine level, and how you say you are feeling,

I don't want to go onto dialysis. The restrictions to my life are more than I'm willing to take. I'm 43 and I've known this day has been coming. Am I wrong? As it stands now, the doctors estimate my kidneys will last maybe a year. Can I have a transplant before I need dialysis?

A kidney transplant is the best form of treatment for ESRF for some people (only 30–40% of patients are 'fit enough' for a transplant). It is a much more effective treatment than dialysis for removing the symptoms of kidney failure. This is because – if it works perfectly – a transplanted kidney can provide up to 50% of the function of two normal kidneys, whereas any type of dialysis can only be equal to 5%.

While you are not wrong in being unwilling to have dialysis, it may still be unwise to refuse it. Dialysis does at least work. Also, the main objective of dialysis, in a person fit enough for a transplant, is to keep them alive long enough for doctors to be able to organise one. If you refuse dialysis, you will die and not get a transplant. Not that a transplant is a cure for kidney failure. Doctors still consider you to be in ESRF, even if you have a transplant. And transplants have their own problems. They do not last forever and it may be necessary for a patient to have a second transplant or to resume dialysis (see Chapter 5 for more about the limitations of transplants).

If a friend or relative is able and willing to donate you one of their kidneys, you may well be able to have a transplant sooner rather than later. Some units can organise cadaveric transplants (transplants from a person who has died) before dialysis. They usually try to do this when the creatinine is over 500 micromoles per litre (less than 10% function). At this point, dialysis is usually necessary within six months. It is quite difficult to 'judge it right' – ie, do a transplant (a major operation) when you are near to 'needing it' but not years before you need it. Other units think it fairer to do a cadaveric transplant after you have started dialysis – so that there is the same 'starting point' for all patients.

I am on haemodialysis. I've heard the phrase 'ESRF'. What does it stand for, and do I have it?

ESRF means 'end-stage renal (kidney) failure'. It is quite difficult to define. The definition has nothing to do with the amount of urine you pass. It is considered to begin when treatment by dialysis or a transplant begins. So, if you have ESRF, you will always have it, no matter what type of dialysis you are on, or if you ever get a transplant. It really means a state in which kidney function is so poor that either dialysis or transplant is essential to keep you alive. In other words, without dialysis or a transplant, you would die.

When kidneys reach 'end-stage' and you are on dialysis, they rarely get better. In a few patients they get better for a while, and dialysis can be stopped for a while, only to be restarted later.

Three hours of haemodialysis is quite enough to cope with. Will I always need the same amount?

The symptoms of kidney failure will tend to worsen if you are under-dialysed, that is if insufficient dialysis is given to bring the blood creatinine down to target levels. This is especially likely to happen in larger, more muscular people, who tend to need more dialysis than those who are smaller. It can also occur in a person of any size at around a year after the start of dialysis. This is because, around this time, the patient's 'own 5%' of kidney function (from their own kidneys) will disappear. This is called the 'loss of residual renal function'.

At this point most patients will notice they pass less urine (and some will pass no urine at all). There are some (fortunate) patients who continue to pass their own '5%' indefinitely. This urine is useful in that it helps to clear water from the body (so they can drink more than other patients). But it is unlikely to clear much in the way of waste products, so the amount of dialysis may still have to be increased. Therefore you may need an increase to three and a half, or even four, hours of haemodialysis a year after starting dialysis – sorry.

The same is also true for PD patients. They may need an increase in the size or number of bags after one year of dialysis.

If I have to have dialysis, do all units give you a free choice between haemodialysis and PD? Which is better anyway?

Some patients are more suitable for one type of dialysis than the other (see pages 91–92). Where this is not the case, however, not many renal units in the UK are able to give patients free choice. In many areas, stretched dialysis resources may limit the availability of haemodialysis. Where this is the case, it will be the people who are unsuitable for PD (for medical or social reasons) who will be prioritised for haemodialysis treatment.

Neither treatment is clearly better than the other, but some patients are more suited for one treatment than the other.

Do I get a free choice between dialysis and a transplant?

No. Only 30–40% of patients are suitable for a transplant. And not all the patients who are suitable, are suitable all the time. Also, there are not enough kidneys from dead people (where most kidneys come from) available, and this situation is not improving. If you are suitable for a transplant, it is usually better to get a kidney from a friend, partner or relative (a 'living transplant' – see Chapter 6).

I am a 56-year-old diabetic patient and I have been on CAPD for four years. I had a heart attack two years ago. Can I have a kidney transplant?

To have a transplant of any kind, you must be very fit. Unfortunately, most people with diabetes have other problems as well. If you have heart disease, for example, you would probably not be suitable for a transplant. This is because the operation can put a lot of strain on your heart, putting you at serious risk.

Some young people who have diabetes, and are well on dialysis, are suitable for a transplant. However, they will need extra tests to make sure their bodies can cope with the operation.

**My dad has diabetes and is blind. He is unable to leave the
house as his legs are so bad. He has had two heart attacks.
To cap it all, his kidney specialist now says his kidney
function is down to 5%, and he needs dialysis to survive.
He refuses to have it. Is 5% considered failure? The
kidney specialist says he will be dead 'within two weeks' if
he does not come into hospital and start dialysis. Is that
true? I don't want him to die. He is only 47 and has
brought me up by himself. I am 14 years old.**

Yes, 5% is considered failure. In fact, anything below 100% is
considered failure, by doctors. It is not true to say he will live
'two weeks'. It is not that predictable. Having said that, it is likely
he will die within 3–6 months (of kidney failure), if he refuses
dialysis. It may not be a bad thing if he makes that decision. Even
though you don't want him to die, dialysis may not necessarily
prolong his life by much. If it does, it may only do so by a few
months.

So, for example, it may make him live for another nine months,
rather than three months or six months without dialysis. But, the
big but, dialysis can be unpleasant, and is always very hard work.
It also involves having one or more operations, and lots of time in
hospital. So, he (and you) might prefer to spend the last few
months of his life at home and together, saying 'goodbye', and all
the other things that you need to say.

He will die without dialysis, but he may well die with it too. So
it is a very difficult decision. If he has decided not to have
dialysis, you will have to do your best to support him in that
decision. But you will need support too. If you do not have other
family members who can provide it, ask your Dad's consultant or
your GP to put you in touch with a social worker.

4
Investigations and other procedures

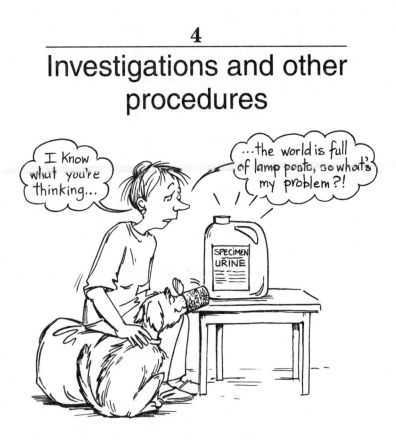

Tests and investigations are a fact of life for people with kidney disease. From the time kidney failure is first suspected, you will find yourself subject to various diagnostic tests. Once it has been established that your kidneys are failing, their condition and yours will need constant monitoring. Further tests will be necessary if you are being considered for a transplant operation.

This chapter gives information about many of the investigations and other procedures you may experience at some time during your life with kidney failure.

Finding out

How do you know if you've got kidney failure?

Although there are many different symptoms of kidney failure, most are non-specific, and could be caused by something else. The only way kidney failure can be diagnosed for certain is by blood and urine tests.

My doctor thinks my kidneys could be failing and has said I will need some tests so that she can be sure. What sort of tests am I likely to have?

If your doctor suspects you have kidney failure, she is likely to order a battery of blood tests. Only one of these, the creatinine test, really matters. If the level of the substance creatinine in your blood is raised (over 120 micromoles is the generally agreed figure), then your kidneys are not working normally. In this case, you will be referred to a local nephrologist (kidney specialist) who will order more blood and urine tests and, as time goes by, some of the other procedures described in the remainder of this chapter.

What is the creatinine clearance? I've been told mine is 10 millilitres per minute? Is this low or high, good or bad? How is it related to the creatinine blood test?

Creatinine clearance is the rate at which the kidneys filter the blood and remove toxins such as creatinine (see above). When the doctor or nurse measures the level of creatinine in your blood they are seeing how much of this waste has built up in the body. The normal level of creatinine in the blood is between 70 and 120 micromoles per litre of blood but this depends on the person's size and muscle bulk. Smaller people (who have smaller muscles) would have less creatinine than bigger people (with bigger muscles). Generally, the lower the level of creatinine in the blood, the better the function of your kidneys.

However, creatinine clearance can be a better gauge of how well the kidneys are functioning because it shows how much creatinine is being removed from the body rather than how much is left. Creatinine clearance is measured by comparing the amount of creatinine in the blood to the amount of creatinine in all the urine (and it must be all the urine) passed in a 24-hour period. The normal rate is approximately 100 millilitres per minute. Unlike the blood creatinine, the higher the level of creatinine clearance the better. So a creatinine clearance of 10 millilitres per minute shows your kidneys are not working very well – the rate of filtration is lower than normal – ie 10%. At this point, the level of creatinine in your blood could be 500 micromoles per litre.

Treatment for kidney failure (dialysis or a transplant) is usually started when the creatinine clearance rate is down to between 5 and 7 % of normal (about 5–7 millilitres per minute) and the blood creatinine has reached more than 600 micromoles per litre.

Dialysis provides a creatinine clearance of at least 5 millilitres per minute (about 5% of normal) and so at the start of dialysis the total creatinine clearance is 10% of what two normal kidneys can do. This includes 5% from dialysis, and 5% residual function from your own kidneys. This is why patients who are treated with dialysis rarely feel 100% well. Ideally, after a transplant the creatinine clearance rate will return to 50% of normal (as you now have one healthy kidney).

Over time, the function of the transplant kidney may improve. How or why this happens is not yet fully understood.

I am on dialysis because I have polycystic kidneys. I've been told this runs in families. Who should be tested in my family?

Polycystic kidney disease (PCKD) tends to run in families, so if you have it the following members of your family should be tested.

(i) **Your parents.** If you have PCKD, it is likely one of your parents also had it, so if they are still alive they should be tested. If they had the disease, their brothers and sisters should also be tested, as should the children of any who test positive.

(ii) **Your brothers and sisters.** If you have PCKD, each of your brothers or sisters has a 50% (1 in 2) chance of having the disease. Men and women have the same chance of having it. If someone is clear of the disease, they cannot pass it on to their children.

(iii) **Your children.** If you have PCKD, each of your children has a 50% chance of having it and should be tested at the appropriate time (see below). The risk is the same for boys and girls.

How do you diagnose PCKD, and when should you have the test?

To find out whether you have polycystic disease, you will need to have an ultrasound scan (see page 85). This is painless and simple.

It is important to know that:

(i) Cysts may not appear in the kidneys until the age of about 20 years. A screening test before this age cannot prove that someone does not have polycystic disease. Therefore, the children of someone with polycystic disease are not usually investigated until they are over 20 years old.

(ii) There is no cure for polycystic disease, no matter how early it is diagnosed. But knowing whether you have it will make it easier for you to plan your life.

(iii) Even though the disease itself is not treatable, some of the complications (such as high blood pressure) will be. So your general level of health may be better if PCKD is diagnosed early and complications can be treated sooner rather than later. In addition, many people would prefer to know in advance if they are likely to develop a serious illness, as they will find it easier to plan their lives. But this is a very personal thing.

Urine tests

**My legs and face started to swell up six weeks ago. My
doctor got me seen at the hospital by a kidney specialist.
He put a small strip of card in my urine and said I had
'nephrotic syndrome'. What was that strip of card, and
how did he know what I had from such a simple test?**

These small strips of card called 'dipsticks' are very clever tests.
They enable doctors and nurses to detect a lot of things in your
urine – blood, protein, sugar, pH (the level of acid). Some strips
also test for white blood cells and nitrites which can indicate an
infection. Normal urine would not contain any blood cells,
protein, sugar or nitrites, and the pH would be acidic at about 6.

Nephrotic syndrome is a problem in which the kidneys' filters
(see pages 7–8) become 'leaky' and start to allow protein to
escape into the urine. Normally, there is almost no protein in the
urine. In severe nephrotic syndrome, up to 10% of the protein you
eat can leak into the urine.

If the dipstick test shows there is a lot of protein in your urine,
this can be a sign of nephrotic syndrome. By itself, the urine test
is not enough to diagnose nephrotic syndrome. Your doctor
would also have taken into account your leg and face swelling.
He probably also had the results of your blood tests, which would
have shown low levels of protein.

There are many different causes of nephrotic syndrome. Your
doctor will probably recommend you have a kidney biopsy (see
pages 82–83). This is the only way of determining the cause. Once
the cause has been discovered, the right treatment can be found
for you.

**My daughter has been admitted to hospital with acute
kidney failure and the nurse has put a urinary catheter
into her bladder. Will this be permanent?**

A urinary catheter is a narrow plastic tube, which goes straight
into the bladder. This is usually done by the nurses on the ward

and can be uncomfortable. Your daughter has been given a urinary catheter so that the urine her kidneys make can be measured accurately. She will only need to have the catheter while her kidneys are not working properly. If she has acute kidney failure (that is, her kidneys stopped working suddenly), there is a good chance the kidneys will get better in a few weeks. There is a small chance your daughter could get an infection from the catheter. If this does happen, it will easily be treated with antibiotics.

I am 36 years old and recently had a medical at work. This detected blood in my urine and I have been referred to a kidney specialist. I have never noticed blood in my urine and I feel fine. Should I worry?

Urine 'dipsticks' (see previous page) are very sensitive to even the smallest drop of blood in your urine. Just because you cannot see any blood, it doesn't mean there isn't any there.

Blood in the urine can be a sign of damage to the kidneys and should always be investigated.

You will probably be sent to see a urologist (a doctor who specialises in bladder, kidney and prostate operations) who will organise an ultrasound and cystoscopy (see pages 82 and 85). If the results of these investigations are normal, you may be sent to see a nephrologist (a doctor who specialises in kidney failure). The nephrologist will take some blood tests and your blood pressure. If all these tests are normal it is unlikely you have a serious problem.

It may be recommended that you continue to have a check-up with the nephrologist once a year.

Why have I been asked to collect all the urine I pass in 24 hours?

You may have had a 'dipstick' urine test (see page 76), which has shown some problems such as protein in your urine. A 24-hour urine collection will show exactly how much protein there is in your urine. It will also enable the laboratory to measure the amount of other substances you are passing such as salt and creatinine (see pages 4–5).

Creatinine is measured so that the doctors and nurses can estimate how well your kidneys are working. They can do this by comparing the amount of creatinine you have in your blood with the amount that you are getting rid of, in your urine. This is called a **creatinine clearance test**. A normal creatinine clearance rate is about 100 millilitres per minute – ie, 100 millilitres of blood is cleared of creatinine every minute, and this cleared creatinine appears in the urine. The higher this number, the better is the kidney function. This is the opposite to blood creatinine which should be lower rather than higher.

When you have a 24-hour urine test, it is absolutely vital you collect every drop of urine you pass in 24 hours. If you miss even one trip to the loo, the test results will be useless.

24-hour urine collections can be more difficult for women to do as men can urinate straight into the bottle.

Blood tests and what they mean

I seem to have an awful lot of blood tests every time I go to clinic. Can you tell me what they are all for?

Measuring the level of various substances in your body is a very important way of finding out how well the dialysis or a transplant is working. The most common tests are to check the levels of waste products (**creatinine** and **urea**), and for salts and other substances.

The normal level of creatinine in the blood is between 70 and 120 micromoles per litre. However, patients who have dialysis will have more creatinine than this because their kidneys are unable to expel it from the body. If you are having peritoneal dialysis (PD), your blood creatinine should be under 800 micromoles per litre. If you have haemodialysis, it should be under 800 micromoles per litre before your dialysis session and 300 micromoles per litre afterwards.

If you have kidney failure, you should know what your creatinine level is at all times.

The salts and other substances monitored by blood tests include **potassium**, **sodium**, **glucose**, **bicarbonate**, **calcium**, **phosphate** and **albumin** (a type of protein).

It is also important to measure levels of **haemoglobin** (or **Hb**) in the blood. This is the substance that carries oxygen around the body. Every part of the body needs a supply of oxygen in order to stay alive. Many patients with kidney failure suffer from **anaemia**, a condition in which there is not enough haemoglobin in the blood to transport the oxygen efficiently. Anaemia causes tiredness, lethargy, breathlessness and poor sex drive.

The normal level of haemoglobin in the blood is 11.7–18 grams per decilitre. If the haemoglobin levels are below this, the patient is said to be anaemic. The level of **ferritin** (which indicates the level of iron) in your blood is also tested as treatments for anaemia will not be effective if this is too low.

The other group of blood tests carried out regularly on patients with kidney failure are called Liver Function Tests (LFTs). These test the levels of various substances:

(i) **Bilirubin.** Levels of this substance indicate how well the liver is working.

(ii) **Aspartate transaminase.** Raised levels indicate that liver cells have been damaged by disease.

(iii) **Alkaline phosphatase.** This test can indicate problems with the drainage of bile, a substance containing the waste products of the liver. It can also alert the doctor to the presence of **renal bone disease** (see pages 59–60).

(iv) **Gamma-glutamyltransferase.** This test also measures how well bile drains from the liver.

A summary of normal and target blood test results for patients on dialysis is given in Appendix 1.

Why does the doctor measure my liver function if I have kidney failure?

The liver is the largest organ in the body and it is found under the rib cage on the right hand side. The liver has many functions, some of which are essential for life.

One of the liver's functions is to destroy the wastes left over from medicines and drugs when they have been used. Some drugs are harmful to the liver and cannot be destroyed. By performing liver function tests, doctors can see whether the drugs you are taking are having a bad effect on your liver.

Some people can get an infection of the liver called hepatitis. There are many different types of hepatitis (including the most common in the UK – hepatitis B and C). The infection can be passed on by infected blood transfusions, during sex, and by drug addicts who share needles for injections.

These days there is very little risk of having an infected blood transfusion as all blood is screened for hepatitis B and C (and HIV, the virus that causes AIDS) before it is given to another patient.

My 19-year-old son has had a blood test that showed creatinine levels of 227 micromoles per litre. What does this mean? His GP has sent a referral letter to a consultant nephrologist, (whatever that is), but after three weeks we have heard nothing further. Should I be concerned and make further enquiries?

Your son's creatinine level is high, and a high level of creatinine in the blood is a sign that the kidneys are not working properly. This is why your GP has sent a referral letter to a consultant nephrologist (a senior doctor who specialises in kidney failure). You should certainly follow this up with your GP to find out the date of your son's appointment with the nephrologist.

Dialysis or a kidney transplant is usually considered for patients who have more than 600 micromoles per litre of creatinine in the blood. The time that it takes for the creatinine to reach this level varies in patients from a few months to many years. For this reason it is very important that your son has the level of creatinine in his blood checked soon, to be sure it is not going up.

I'm a dialysis patient and am in hospital at the moment. Why do the nurses take my blood pressure so often?

Blood pressure is partly controlled by your kidneys (see page 5). It is important that it is monitored regularly so that very low or very high blood pressure can be spotted and treated.

Just measuring your blood pressure once will not give an accurate guide, as it tends to go up and down a lot during the course of a day. Frequent measurement allows the medical team to see what is your average blood pressure. Measuring blood pressure with a manual machine (sphygmomanometer) is unreliable as people use different machines in different ways. The newer, electronic blood pressure machines are more accurate and therefore preferred in many renal units.

My husband has had high blood pressure for a few years. It is always higher when he goes to the hospital than when it is measured at our GP surgery. Is this because he gets stressed when he goes to the hospital?

Blood pressure is unlikely to go up that much in stressful situations. It is more likely your GP is using a different type of machine from that used in the hospital, or taking your husband's blood pressure in a different way.

Your husband may need to have a 24-hour blood pressure test. This uses a small machine attached to a blood pressure cuff placed around the arm. It should be left in place for 24 hours, during which time he should try to behave normally. It will measure his blood pressure every 15 minutes and record it on a small computer so that the doctors can look at it. This will enable them to get a true recording of his average blood pressure.

Other procedures

I am a 43-year-old man. Over the last year, I keep seeing blood in my urine. I have been seen by a hospital specialist called a urologist and he has told me I need a cystoscopy. What does this mean?

A cystoscopy is a simple investigation where a tiny camera is passed up the hole in your penis so that the doctor can see into your bladder. In a woman the camera is passed up the urethra (the tube through which she passes urine). You may be given a general anaesthetic (put to sleep) for the cystoscopy, but many doctors just use a local anaesthetic to do it, and you remain awake during the test.

During the test the doctor will look for kidney stones, cancer or any other abnormalities. It usually takes about 20 minutes and most people can go home the same day.

There are few risks with this investigation, but there is a possibility the camera could make a hole in your bladder. Although this is rare it could be extremely serious.

I have recently been diagnosed with kidney failure and the hospital has sent me for an appointment to have a kidney biopsy. They haven't told me anything else about it and I'm very worried. Please help.

A kidney biopsy is a procedure where a very small piece of kidney is removed so it can be examined under a microscope. This is sometimes the only way for the doctors to tell what is wrong with your kidneys.

A hollow needle, called a biopsy needle, is used to remove two or three samples of your kidney. The sample is taken from the surface of the kidney.

A kidney biopsy is performed on just one of your kidneys (most people have two) because it is assumed that if one of your kidneys is damaged, the other one will be as well. The procedure may be done in the X-ray department, or it might be done on the renal ward.

During the kidney biopsy you will be asked to lie on your front. Before the doctor does the biopsy, he or she will inject some local anaesthetic to numb the skin. You will remain awake throughout the whole procedure. An ultrasound scan (see page 85) will be used to help the doctor to find the exact location of your kidney. Even though the biopsy itself takes only a few seconds, the whole process will take 20 minutes or so.

Afterwards, you will probably be asked to lie flat on your back for 6–12 hours. During this period, the nurses will take your pulse rate and blood pressure regularly. If your pulse rate goes up and/or your blood pressure goes down, this can indicate bleeding (see risks of biopsy, overleaf). You will also be asked to show any urine you pass to the nurse, who will check it for signs of bleeding.

It is usually necessary to stay in hospital overnight. In some hospitals, though, the biopsy is done as 'day surgery', usually first thing in the morning so you can go home in the early evening. This is quite safe as, if complications are going to occur, they will usually do so in the first 2–4 hours after the procedure.

Some results of the biopsy are usually available the same day (if it is done in the morning), or the following day. The full report can take 2–3 weeks to come through.

The kidney biopsy procedure may hurt and you will probably have some pain for up to four weeks afterwards. It is important you take it easy after the biopsy for at least a week. During that week, don't play any sport, do any strenuous activities or have sex. You should also take a week off work.

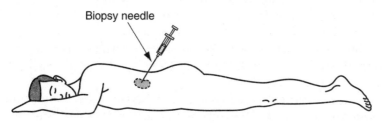

Biopsy needle

Figure 5 Kidney biopsy

Most people only need one biopsy in their lifetime. Some people need several, especially if they have had a kidney transplant (see pages 144–146).

Are there any risks involved in having a kidney biopsy?

The most common problem with a kidney biopsy is that the doctor is unable to get a sample of the kidney. This happens in about one in every 20 biopsies performed. If the doctor can't get the sample, you will probably have to have another biopsy on another day.

The other risk after a kidney biopsy is from bleeding. About one in every 100 people who have a kidney biopsy suffer from a bleeding kidney afterwards. This means you will have blood in your urine. It usually gets better on its own. However, very rarely (in about one in 1,000 cases) a patient can bleed so badly that the kidney will need to be removed, in an emergency operation. If this happens to you it might mean you will need dialysis earlier than expected. In very rare cases, the bleeding can be so severe as to be life-threatening.

I had a transplant operation four weeks ago, the kidney is not working very well, and I am still in hospital. I run my own business and I need to go back to work. I am beginning to regret having it. I have had to have a kidney biopsy every week for the last four weeks. Is this safe? Will it help the kidney to work?

A kidney biopsy for a transplant kidney is similar to a biopsy of your own kidney (see page 82). But there are a few differences. You will be asked to lie on your back during the procedure because the transplanted kidney has been put into the front of your abdomen (see pages 138–139). Should the biopsy cause so much bleeding that the kidney has to be removed, you will have to go back onto dialysis immediately.

It is quite common to have several biopsies following a transplant, as this is the only way the doctors can find out if your body is rejecting the kidney. Performing the biopsy should not damage the kidney but it will not help it to work better either.

The risks of a transplant biopsy are similar to those of a biopsy of your own kidneys.

I have early kidney failure but I am not yet on dialysis. My doctor has asked me to have ultrasound scan. Please can you tell me why?

An ultrasound scan is a test that can see any organ inside your body by using sound waves. It is common for pregnant women to have ultrasound scans to look at their unborn baby.

An ultrasound scan of the kidneys is normally performed in the X-ray department although some renal wards have their own machine. A special jelly is spread on the skin and an ultrasound probe is moved over the abdomen, allowing the kidneys to be seen on the screen. The doctor can see if your kidneys are shrunken, enlarged or even missing. An ultrasound scan can also show whether there are any problems, such as blockages, in the tubes that take urine from your kidneys to your bladder.

Ultrasound is often used to help find the cause of kidney failure. In some patients, for example those with polycystic kidneys (see pages 19–20), it can actually make a diagnosis. In other patients, for example those with renovascular disease (see pages 15–16), it can be used along with other tests to make a diagnosis. It may also be done as part of another test. For example it may be used during a kidney biopsy (see page 82) or nephrostomy (see page 89) to help the doctor to find out exactly where your kidneys are.

The scan itself is usually painless. This is because it uses a small probe that sends sound waves around the body and sound waves do not hurt. Also, the ultrasound does not pierce the body. The pattern of the sound waves that return to the probe allows the machine to form a picture of what the kidneys look like. If appropriate, the person carrying out the test may print photographs of certain images seen on the screen. It takes about 10–15 minutes to carry out an ultrasound test of the kidneys.

I have had many ultrasound scans of my kidneys recently (I have just had a transplant) and last time the machine made a loud whooshing noise. Was the ultrasound machine faulty?

It sounds as though you had a 'Doppler test' at the same time as your ultrasound scan. This test is used to check the amount of blood flowing into and out of your new kidney. If you heard a whooshing noise, that is usually a good sign.

I have been told I need to have an ultrasound scan to help the doctors find out why I have kidney failure. I received the appointment yesterday and it's not for another four months. I am very worried about my diagnosis – is there any way that it could be done sooner?

Your ultrasound scan is very important as it will help the doctors to find out why your kidneys are not working and therefore give you the most appropriate treatment. There is no point going to see your doctor again until the results of the scan are known.

In many parts of the UK waiting for investigations can take a long time and is frustrating for both the patients and the medical team. There is little you can do, but you could try calling your doctor and telling him that your test is not for four months. He may be able to get the date brought forward. Unfortunately, the X-ray department will not be able to do this for you.

I need to have a renal angiogram. What does this involve and what will it tell the doctor?

A renal angiogram is an X-ray picture of the main blood vessel that goes to a kidney from the heart (ie, the renal artery). It is done to look at either the main blood vessel to a person's own kidney, or to a transplant kidney, and can help the doctors to determine whether there is a blockage in the renal artery. This can be a cause of high blood pressure or kidney failure.

The procedure can be performed either on a day case basis (you arrive, have the test, and leave, on the same day) or it may require an overnight stay in hospital. Angiograms are usually done in the X-ray department. A specialist X-ray doctor will numb your groin with a local anaesthetic injection. Then a thin tube is passed into the femoral artery (a blood vessel in your groin). This plastic tube is fed up the artery towards the kidney. In the case of a transplant angiogram, the transplant artery is lower down, and comes off the leg artery so the catheter does not have to go as far. A special dye, which can be seen on an X-ray, is injected through the tube. This will show the doctor if there are any blockages in the blood vessel.

If a blockage is found, the doctor can remove it by inflating a small balloon at the end of the tube, which will flatten the blockage. This is called an angioplasty.

As with many procedures, there are some risks with an angiogram. These include bruising in the groin, which is very common, and pain. The X-ray dye is toxic to kidneys and so may damage them. There is a 5% risk that this will make your kidney function worse, but this can be as high as 10% if you have diabetes or a degree of kidney failure before the test. There is a 2% chance of the dye causing your kidney so much damage that you will need dialysis earlier than expected. Occasionally, people are allergic to the dye and get a nasty reaction. An angiogram can be fatal in a very small proportion of cases (about one in a thousand for a renal angiogram, but possibly rising to as much as one in a hundred if angioplasty is attempted).

My doctor has suggested I have a CT scan, but I am not keen. Please tell me why I should have it. I have already had an ultrasound.

A Computerised Tomography (CT) scan is a type of X-ray. It does not hurt and usually only takes about 10 minutes. The machine used for a CT scan is a very large tube which some patients find claustrophobic.

CT scans enable the doctor to get a detailed picture of the kidney without cutting you open. Sometimes a special dye can be injected into a vein in your arm to help the doctor see more clearly. This dye is toxic and can make your kidney function worse. Occasionally, people are allergic to the dye and get a reaction which can be fatal.

These days, CT scans are not done very often because ultrasound scans are sufficiently detailed in most cases. There are still a few circumstances however where a CT scan provides additional detail to an ultrasound scan.

My GP thinks my kidney function is bad. He has referred me to the local hospital for a test called an IVP. Please could you give me more information about this test?

An IVP (intravenous pyleogram) is another type of X-ray. A special dye that can be seen inside your body on an X-ray is injected into a vein in your arm. As the dye travels around your body, the doctor looks to see where it goes. This can help him or her to see if there are any blockages, such as kidney stones, in your kidneys and their drainage tubes (see page 7).

This dye is toxic and can make your kidney function worse. It can also cause an allergic reaction in a few people, which can be fatal. It rarely gives clear pictures if kidney failure is severe.

I have had lots of investigations to try to find the cause of my kidney failure. The doctor has now asked me to go for a nuclear medicine scan. This sounds quite risky – will I get radiation poisoning?

A nuclear medicine scan uses an injection of radioactive dye to make a detailed picture of your kidneys. The level of radioactivity is very low and not harmful. This type of scan is quite common because it is very safe.

The test takes place in the nuclear medicine department of the hospital.

There are two types of nuclear medicine scan. The first, a **DMSA** scan, is used to look for scars in the kidney. The second, a **DTPA** (or **MAG3**) scan, can be used to see how well each kidney is working. Another use is to look for obstruction to the drainage of urine from the kidneys to the bladder.

My father is in hospital with severe kidney failure. He has been told that his kidneys are blocked. What can be done to help?

Your father will probably have a procedure called a **nephrostomy** carried out very soon.

A specialist X-ray doctor will do this in the X-ray department. Your father will not be put to sleep but will have some local anaesthetic to numb the pain. The doctor will use an ultrasound scan (see page 85) to make sure he knows the exact location of the blocked kidney. A thin plastic tube will then be passed through the site of your father's abdomen, into the centre of the kidney. This tube will be left in place so that any urine the kidney makes can be drained through the tube and out of his body. A special plastic bag will be attached to the end of the tube to collect all the urine.

There is a small chance that the plastic tube used in the nephrostomy can cause the kidney to bleed. If the bleeding is very bad, the kidney may need to be removed during an operation. If this happens, your father may need dialysis, perhaps for the rest of his life. There is also a small risk of death if the bleeding is severe.

However, if he does not have the nephrostomy, the kidney will stay blocked and this will cause permanent damage to the kidney. If both kidneys are blocked and nothing is done, your father will almost certainly need dialysis. If both kidneys are blocked, he is likely to need a nephrostomy in each one. These will be done on separate days.

What is an MRI scan?

MRI stands for **Magnetic Resonance Imaging**. This is a special type of scan that shows the kidneys in close detail.

If you have a pacemaker, an MRI scan can be dangerous, so you should be sure that your doctor knows if you do have one. Also, alert the doctor if you have any metal inside your body, such as a hip replacement or metal plate in your leg. It may affect the quality of the image or, in some cases, ruin the scan.

5
Dialysis

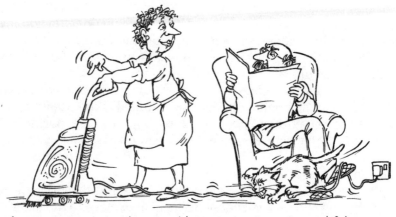

"Yes, Mrs. B. — I too would like something 'wiv a lifetime filter an' no bag changes'... a new kidney, in fact!"

Dialysis is a process by which waste and excess water is removed from the blood. This is the most important function normally carried out by the kidneys, but if they have failed it needs to be done artificially.

There are two types of dialysis, **peritoneal dialysis (PD)** and **haemodialysis**. In both processes, the blood is filtered to remove creatinine, urea, other wastes and excess water, while keeping the important parts of the blood such as blood cells and nutrients.

Introduction to dialysis

I am about to start something called PD. It doesn't sound like proper dialysis. What is it?

PD is short for 'peritoneal dialysis'. It certainly is proper dialysis, but is only one of the two types of dialysis available.

PD uses a part of the body, the **peritoneum**, as a filter. The peritoneum is a natural membrane that lines the inside of the abdominal wall and covers all the abdominal organs (the stomach, bowels, liver, etc.). It resembles a balloon in appearance and texture but has lots of tiny holes which enable it to be used as a dialysis membrane. As blood flows through the blood vessels in the peritoneum, water and toxins easily pass through the holes, but blood cells are too large.

The peritoneum has two layers – one lining the inside of the abdominal wall, the other lining the abdominal organs. Between these two layers is a space. This space is called the **peritoneal cavity**. During PD, it is the peritoneal cavity that is used as a reservoir for the dialysis fluid. Normally, the peritoneal cavity contains only about 100 ml of liquid. However, as women who have been pregnant know, it can expand to hold up to 5 litres of liquid.

The other type of dialysis, haemodialysis, uses a **dialysis machine** and an **artificial kidney** to remove excess water from the body. A process known as ultrafiltration or 'u f ing' creates a negative pressure through the machine. This is known as transmembrane pressure, or TMP, and it causes water to be sucked from the blood.

I am 42 and need to start dialysis soon. Which should I have, PD or haemodialysis?

As a general rule, you will be suitable for most therapy options most of the time. In fact, you may experience every therapy – PD, haemodialysis and transplant – at some point in your life. It is very unlikely that one treatment will never be suitable for you, however there are times when one could be more suitable for you than another.

As a first treatment option, peritoneal dialysis is often more suitable for a number of reasons. If your kidneys are still working, no matter how little, they may carry on working for longer with PD. If you have diabetes, you may also have weak veins. As your veins are needed in order to perform haemodialysis, it is sensible not to damage them early in your life on dialysis. By having PD first, you can 'save' your veins so they can be used in later years when PD may no longer be effective.

PD is a home therapy, whereas most patients who have haemodialysis are treated in hospital. Many people who are just starting dialysis prefer to be treated at home rather than making frequent trips to the hospital.

Will dialysis make me better? Will I ever be cured?

Dialysis will not 'cure' you, or anyone with kidney failure. It cannot get rid of the symptoms completely, or restore your kidneys to health. What it can do, however, is control your symptoms and stop you from dying.

The symptoms of kidney failure never really go away because PD or haemodialysis can provide only about 5% of the function of two normal kidneys. So when you start dialysis, you will usually have only about 10% of the function of two normal kidneys (5% from dialysis, and 5% from your own kidneys). This is simply not enough.

Even though dialysis technology has its limitations, it does exist and it does work. So it is sensible to start treatment as early as possible – before you become very unwell. The doctor will be able to tell from your blood creatinine and symptoms when is the best time to start dialysis.

Can you have too much dialysis, or be 'over dialysed'?

There is no such thing as too much dialysis. This is because dialysis can realistically provide around 5% of the function of two normal kidneys. Even if a patient were to have haemodialysis seven days a week this would still not reach the level of normal kidney function. As a rule, it is best to have the maximum amount of dialysis possible without infringing on your lifestyle.

What is the best type of dialysis for elderly patients?

There is no 'best treatment' for older people. It depends on your lifestyle, your health and what treatment you prefer.

If you still like a lot of freedom to travel, PD gives you the chance to do this with a minimum of fuss and organisation. It is possible you would feel fitter on PD because, in some elderly patients, the heart and blood vessels are not as strong and flexible as they were when they were younger. This may make haemodialysis uncomfortable because, being an intermittent treatment (three times a week), a large amount of fluid is removed over a short period of time during dialysis. This may put a strain on the heart, which may already be working less well than it should, and can make you feel 'washed out' or faint.

PD is a gentler treatment because you are receiving dialysis continuously, removing excess fluid slowly and at a steady rate. This is kinder to the body, which does not have to adjust to sudden changes. If, however, you are getting frail and dependent on others, it may be difficult to perform the exchanges. If you have arthritic hands, difficulty seeing, or problems with carrying and lifting heavy bags, you might prefer to have your treatment done for you. For this reason, most frail elderly patients are treated in hospital with haemodialysis. These patients are often widowed or living alone, and actually welcome the visits to hospital, because they get out of the house three times a week and meet other people.

Peritoneal dialysis (PD)

I am about to start peritoneal dialysis. What will happen?

To receive PD, you will need a small operation, which will be performed using local or general anaesthetic. During this, a

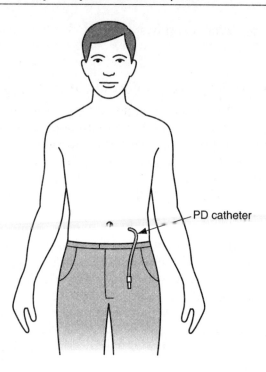

PD catheter

Figure 6 Position of PD catheter

plastic tube will be permanently inserted into your abdomen. This tube is called a PD catheter. It is about 30 cm (12 in) long and as wide as a pencil.

Your PD catheter will be placed through the lower abdominal wall, into the peritoneal cavity. Half of the catheter lies inside your abdomen, and half lies outside. It comes out on the right or the left, under your navel (tummy button). The PD catheter acts as a permanent pathway into your peritoneal cavity from the outside world. It is your dialysis 'lifeline'.

You should be allowed to go home one or two days after the operation. Your catheter is usually 'left alone' for five days or more after the operation before it can be used for dialysis. This allows it to 'settle in' and gives the abdominal wound time to heal.

How does the tube stay in?

The catheter is made from a soft plastic and has two Dacron (felt) cuffs part way down the length of the tube. The first of these cuffs is placed just beneath the skin. The second is placed just outside the peritoneal cavity, deep inside the abdomen. These cuffs 'grow' into the body holding it in place. They also provide a seal to prevent germs entering the body, and the fluid from leaking out.

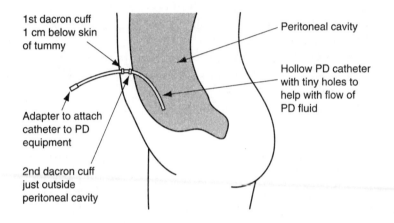

1st dacron cuff
1 cm below skin
of tummy

Peritoneal cavity

Hollow PD catheter
with tiny holes to
help with flow of
PD fluid

Adapter to attach
catheter to PD
equipment

2nd dacron cuff
just outside
peritoneal cavity

Figure 7 The PD catheter in position

My doctor says I must have an operation to have a PD catheter inserted. What is the success rate of operations like this?

Inserting a PD catheter may seem like a simple operation, but in fact it is quite complicated. The success rate is only 70–80%, even with an experienced surgeon. If you have had previous surgery in the tummy, especially low down (in the pelvis), the success rate can be as low as 20–30%. If it can be predicted that the operation will be difficult, you may be advised to go for haemodialysis instead.

What does CAPD stand for?

This form of PD is 'Continuous' and 'Ambulatory', ie 'while you walk around'. Patients walk around with the dialysis fluid in their abdomen. At the end of each period of dialysis, they have to change the dialysis fluid themselves.

When patients are on CAPD, they do their own fluid exchanges. They drain 1.5 to 3 litres of dialysis fluid into their abdomen, leave it there for four to eight hours, and then drain it out. This is done four to five times a day – every day. It is as simple as that. With practice, an exchange of fluid can be done in about 20–30 minutes. Exchanges are simple to do and can be performed almost anywhere.

The dialysis fluid is kept in sealed plastic bags. The bags are connected and disconnected to the peritoneal catheter with a system of tubes and clamps.

What is APD?

APD stands for Automated Peritoneal Dialysis. APD uses a machine to do the dialysis fluid exchanges for you. The machine (which is likely to be about the size of a video recorder) is usually placed at your bedside and does the exchanges while you are asleep.

Most patients need to spend eight to ten hours attached to the machine every night. This enables the machine to perform an average of six exchanges of 1.5 to 3 litres of dialysis fluid each night. The length of time that PD fluid is left in the abdomen before it is exchanged by the machine varies from between about 30 minutes and three hours. After spending the night on the machine, most people on APD keep fluid inside their peritoneum during the daytime without needing to exchange it.

There is no need to have a helper to assist with APD unless you are unable to perform the treatment on your own.

Which is better, CAPD or APD?

In most renal units in the UK, about 60% of the PD patients currently do CAPD and 40% do APD. However, the number of patients doing APD is growing all the time. Different patients may be better suited to either treatment, for a number of reasons.

- **How the peritoneum works**
  The main medical reason why a doctor may choose either CAPD or APD for a patient relates to the way the patient's peritoneum works during dialysis. Some patients, known as 'high transporters', have a peritoneum which works best with more frequent exchanges of dialysis fluid. High transporters are usually more suited to APD, because the machine is able to do rapid exchanges of dialysis fluid while they sleep. Other patients, called 'low transporters', will get more dialysis if the fluid is left inside them for longer periods. Low transporters are generally better suited to CAPD.

  A test has been developed to find out whether patients are 'high' or 'low transporters'. This test is called a Peritoneal Equilibration Test, or PET, and is usually performed in hospital by a nurse. It takes four hours to complete and involves doing just one CAPD exchange. The test measures how quickly the toxins move out of the patient's bloodstream and into the dialysis fluid. If the toxins move quickly, the patient is called a 'high transporter'. If the toxins move slowly, the patient is a 'low transporter'.

- **Patient size**
  APD can be particularly good for patients who require a lot of dialysis – for example, large people, especially those who no longer pass urine. This is because the machine can do more fluid exchanges than patients are able to do themselves with CAPD. Also, as the patients are lying down, they may be more able to tolerate bigger volumes of dialysis fluid. In these ways, APD can remove more waste toxins than CAPD. Even so, for some very large patients, APD during the night may not be enough. Such patients commonly need an additional CAPD exchange at tea-time.

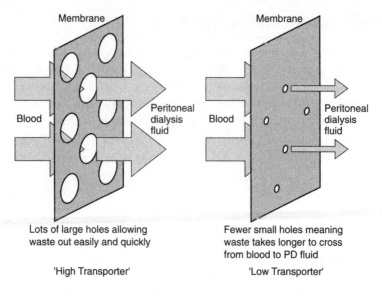

Figure 8 'High transporters' and 'Low transporters'
(*left*) People with bigger holes in their peritoneal membranes
are more suited to APD
(*right*) People with smaller holes in their peritoneal membranes
are more suited to CAPD

- **Patients with a carer**
  APD is a possible treatment option for patients who need a carer to perform dialysis for them, such as the elderly, infirm or very young.

- **Employment reasons**
  Since APD exchanges are done during the night, this form of dialysis can be particularly suitable for people in full-time work or education.

Do all units give you a free choice between CAPD and APD?

Many renal units in the UK are not able to offer a choice between CAPD and APD initially, due to a lack of money. Most renal units will give patients APD eventually. Patients who are medically or socially more suited may be given preference for APD.

Will my diet be restricted when I start PD?

PD is a continuous treatment. It works at removing excess waste products and water from your body 24 hours a day seven days a week, whereas haemodialysis is done intermittently, three times a week for 3–5 hours. For this reason, the excess wastes and water you consume are being continually removed by PD. Unlike patients on haemodialysis, you will have few restrictions on your diet.

What are the complications of being on peritoneal dialysis?

The most common complication of PD is infection (see page 100). However, most infections can be prevented with the proper care and attention to cleanliness, and are easily treated.

You may also suffer from constipation. This can cause problems with the drainage of the dialysis fluid and so it is important to avoid it. If your doctor prescribes laxatives, you should take them regularly to prevent constipation.

Fluid overload is another common problem. The amount of 'used' fluid drained out of the body after PD is about 1.5 litres per day more than the amount of fresh dialysis fluid that is put in. This extra fluid – in effect, the patient's urine – does not increase in quantity however much the patient drinks. To avoid problems due to fluid overload, therefore, most patients need to limit the amount they drink to about 1500 millilitres (just under 3 pints) a day.

The pressure of fluid inside the abdomen sometimes causes problems such as back pain and hernias. Hernias occur when a small section of the muscle wall weakens, allowing part of the bowel to protrude and form a lump in the tummy. Exercising the abdominal and back muscles to keep them strong may help you prevent both of these problems, but if you do suffer from either, you should see your doctor.

I have been asked to collect all the PD fluid I drain out in 24 hours and all the urine I pass. I then have to take all this into the hospital. It seems an awful lot of mess and effort and nobody will tell me what I'm doing it for.

The reason you have been asked to do this is so that your creatinine clearance can be measured accurately now you are on dialysis. The creatinine excreted by your kidneys can be measured in the urine. Creatinine removed by dialysis can be measured in the PD fluid you drain out. These two measurements are added together and compared to the level of creatinine in your blood. This shows how effectively the wastes from your body are being removed. Your creatinine clearance should be at least 70 litres a week. In other words, PD should be clearing the toxin from 70 litres of blood in a week.

When I drain my dialysis fluid out it looks cloudy. Should I be worried?

Cloudy dialysis fluid almost always indicates you have an infection called **peritonitis**. You may well have pain and a temperature too. Peritonitis can be serious but, if it is caught early and treated properly, it is usually not too much of a problem.

Peritonitis is an infection of the peritoneal membrane. It is usually caused by one of two types of germ (*Staphylococcus epidermidis* or *Staphylococcus aureus*). These germs are usually harmless and live on your skin. They only cause a problem when they get inside your body. In rare but serious cases, peritonitis in PD patients is caused by a fungus (usually a type called *Candida albicans*).

The most common route for these germs to enter your body is through the dialysis catheter. This usually happens during the exchange procedure, when the fluid bags are connected to the catheter. However, germs entering the body via the catheter exit site can also cause peritonitis. It is important to follow all the procedures you are taught by the nurses, and pay strict attention to cleanliness.

Germs entering the peritoneum from inside your own body (say from the bowel wall) sometimes cause peritonitis. This is common in people with diverticular disease. Diverticular disease is caused by small pieces of digested food getting caught in the inside of the bowel wall. Peritonitis infections originating inside the body cannot be prevented by cleanliness, but some patients with diverticular disease may be helped by having parts of affected bowel removed in an operation.

The treatment for most types of peritonitis is simple and effective – usually one or more antibiotics to be added to the fresh dialysis fluid. You will be shown how to do this so you can treat yourself at home. If your peritonitis is caused by *Candida albicans*, your catheter will probably need to be removed and a new one put in when you have recovered from the infection.

The area around my PD catheter has become red and itchy. What should I do?

This area is called the exit site and is prone to infection if it is not looked after carefully. Signs of exit site infection are red and itchy skin, bleeding or a yellowy discharge. If you leave it untreated, an exit site infection can become very troublesome and cause serious problems such as peritonitis. Treatment is usually a course of antibiotics and it is important you take the whole course prescribed.

There are a number of effective ways to prevent exit site infections. Most important is making sure that your catheter and tubing is always firmly secured to your skin. This can be done using special tape. It is also important to keep your exit site clean and dry. You may be asked to change the dressing covering the catheter every day. If the dressing becomes wet or dislodged it must be changed as soon as possible.

Can I have a transplant if I have peritonitis?

You will not be offered a transplant if a kidney becomes available for you during an attack of peritonitis. This is because the drugs you are given after a transplant to prevent kidney rejection may make the peritonitis worse. These drugs, called immuno-suppressants, make it harder for the body's immune (defence) system to fight any type of invader (including germs as well as transplanted organs).

Will my PD catheter ever have to be removed?

It is rare for a PD catheter to be removed. The most common reason for taking the tube out is if you have a successful transplant, when it is no longer needed. It could also be removed if your kidneys started working again, but this is extremely rare.

If you got a very bad attack of peritonitis, say that did not clear up after seven days of antibiotics, or if it was caused by *Candida albicans*, your catheter might have to be removed. Other reasons for removing the catheter would be if you had an exit site infection which did not clear up, or if you got repeated attacks of peritonitis. In most cases it is necessary to remove the catheter and wait for the infection to clear up, before inserting a new one. In the meantime, haemodialysis would be necessary. Occasionally, it is possible to insert a new catheter, at the same operation in which the old one is removed. This is sometimes called an 'out-in'.

Your catheter would also need to be removed if it were damaged, cut or punctured. This can happen if for example, you use scissors near the tube. Sometimes the tube can be repaired but, depending on the location of the damage, it may be necessary to replace the catheter. This can be done at the same time the catheter is removed.

How will I be trained to do PD? Do I need to provide any equipment?

You will be taught how to do your PD by qualified and experienced PD nurses. You will either be taught in your renal unit, at home or in a special training centre. You will probably have this training a week or so after your PD catheter operation. You will receive a lot of support and care from the nursing staff during your treatment.

You will not have to provide any equipment yourself.

Before you are expected to carry out your own dialysis, specialist nurses will train you in all aspects of your care. Most patients can become competent in the exchange technique in 3–14 days. When patients first go home after training and have to do the exchanges by themselves, they may find it a bit daunting. However, the nurses will always be available to provide advice and information on the telephone. Most patients find they are doing the dialysis by themselves with no problems within a few weeks.

What if I can't learn how to do it properly, or if there is a problem? Is there anyone who can come and help me?

PD is easy to learn and most patients learn how to do it in a week or so. However, there are some people who cannot do the dialysis themselves for a variety of reasons. You may have a physical problem, such as arthritis in your hands, that means that you can't do the exchanges, or you may simply be too frail.

In these circumstances you might need help from a friend or relative. Then, APD may be the best option. The helper can set the machine up and put you on it at night, then not have to worry until the next morning. They can then take you off the machine and dispose of the used equipment.

Most renal units provide a 24-hour back-up service, whereby a nurse or technician can be called on for advice or to visit your home if there are difficulties. Some nursing homes will also offer to train staff so they can do the dialysis for the patient.

If you are on APD and the machine goes wrong in the middle of the night, the first thing you should do is disconnect yourself from it. You can call your unit back-up service or the manufacturer's helpline (the makers of some APD machines provide these on a 24-hour basis). If necessary, they may provide a replacement machine within six hours of a fault being reported.

If CAPD is the only option for the patient, the carer would need to be very committed as they would need to do the dialysis four times a day, every day.

How often will I need to come to hospital when I'm on PD?

You should have regular check ups in hospital every two to three months when you are on PD. The PD nurses may also visit you occasionally at home or at work. However, if you have any problems between routine check ups, you should contact the renal unit immediately.

I don't like the idea of having tubes sticking out of my body. What can I do to make myself look as normal as possible?

Some PD patients do not like the way dialysis affects their appearance. The abdomen tends to get stretched by PD, giving it a rounded appearance. Young people in particular may be conscious of their body shape, especially if they are slim. Keeping fit and doing exercises to strengthen the abdominal muscles will help.

The PD catheter can also cause body image problems. Patients have to come to terms with the fact that they now have a plastic tube permanently protruding from their abdomen. Some people find this difficult to cope with. They may also worry that the catheter might put off a sexual partner.

Sexual problems – such as reduced sex drive, impotence, and problems with fertility – are common among people with kidney failure. Not all kidney patients have sexual problems, however, and a range of treatments is available for those who do. More information about living and loving positively with PD can be found in Chapter 7.

Why are there different types of fluid used in PD?

For both CAPD and APD, dialysis solution or fluid is used. The ability to remove toxins can be raised by increasing either the volume of fluid used, or the number of exchanges, or both. A larger bag will remove more toxins (and a little more water) than a smaller bag. The dialysis needs of patients depend partly on their body size. Big people usually need 'big bags' (2.5 or 3 litres of dialysis fluid).

The ability of PD fluid to remove water is affected by the amount of glucose (sugar) in the bag – the more glucose in the bag, the more water is removed. There are three different strengths: a 'strong' bag (3.86% glucose solution), a 'medium' bag (2.27% glucose) and a 'weak' bag (1.36% glucose).

The strength of the bag does not relate to its size. A strong bag has more glucose in it than a weak bag, but is no larger. Patients are advised to consider the weak bag as their 'standard' bag, and to try to use a minimum number of strong bags.

There are a number of 'special' dialysis fluids, which are sometimes prescribed for patients with particular problems.

(i) **Icodextrin**

This fluid contains a glucose polymer (in which the glucose molecules are stuck together), rather than ordinary glucose. Icodextrin may be recommended for PD patients who are diabetic or overweight. This is because the glucose polymer in Icodextrin is less likely than ordinary glucose to be absorbed into the body to cause problems with sugar balance or weight gain. Icodextrin is also good at removing excess fluid from patients when it is left in the peritoneum for a long time, for example overnight in CAPD patients, or during the day in APD patients. It has also been shown to benefit patients who have been on PD for a long time and whose peritoneums do not work very well for dialysis.

(ii) **Amino acids**

Some dialysis fluids use amino acids rather than glucose. Amino acids are the building blocks of protein. Some of the amino acids are absorbed into the blood. It is thought these dialysis fluids might also act as food supplements and be particularly useful for patients who are malnourished.

(iii) **Bicarbonate**

A bicarbonate-based dialysis fluid has been developed to help patients who have problems regulating the level of acid in their bodies. This solution may also be good for people who experience pain when the fluid is drained in.

How do I get supplies for PD at home?

The bags of dialysis fluid come in boxes of four or five, so a month's supplies can be as many as 40 boxes. You will also need many other products for PD, such as cleaning fluid and dressings. These can all be stored in a cupboard under the stairs, a spare bedroom, a shed or even a garage.

Most people receive a delivery of supplies once a month, though patients with small houses or flats may be able to arrange fortnightly deliveries. The people who deliver the supplies deliver to many other dialysis patients and are specially recruited and trained to go into patients' homes. They will move the supplies to exactly where you want them, and will even move boxes around so that fluid from previous deliveries gets used before the new stock.

Can I have PD if I have diabetes?

PD is a good treatment option for people with diabetes – indeed many doctors think it is better than haemodialysis. But most patients will absorb a little glucose or sugar (between 100 and 150 grams or 4–6 ounces per day) from their dialysis solution, which can lead to problems. If just one of the glucose solution bags is substituted for an alternative solution, such as the icodextrin or amino acid solution described above, the amount of glucose the patient absorbs will be reduced.

It seems to take me forever to drain the fluid out of my tummy. Sometimes an exchange can take over two hours. Why is this and is there anything I can do to speed things up?

There appears to be a drainage problem with your catheter. The most likely reason for this is constipation. If you become constipated, your bowels press against the catheter and make the dialysis fluid drain very slowly. The fluid may also get trapped in pockets of bowel, preventing it from draining properly. So, it is very important to avoid constipation. Many doctors recommend regular laxatives for all CAPD patients to keep their bowels working well.

It is possible too that your PD catheter might have become blocked with a substance called fibrin. This is a form of protein which looks like tiny strands of cotton wool and is completely harmless. You may be able to clear the catheter simply by squeezing the tubing to dislodge the fibrin. Alternatively, a nurse will be able to clear it by injecting water, saline or a de-clotting agent, called heparin, down the catheter. This is a simple procedure and will not need an operation.

Another reason for poor drainage might be that your catheter is in the wrong position. The tip of your catheter should be quite low down inside your tummy, pointing towards your feet. Sometimes a displaced catheter will 'float' back into the right position naturally. If this does not happen, a small operation may be required to correct the position of the catheter.

Whatever the cause of poor drainage, you should try to get the problem solved, because the time you take to drain out the fluid is 'lost' time – you will not be receiving dialysis while you have little or no fluid in the peritoneum. In addition, such a long drainage time will seriously affect the quality of your life. You should not have to put up with this.

I have been on CAPD for a few months now and I woke up this morning to find that my testicles were really swollen. Could this problem be connected to my CAPD? I'm too embarrassed to go to the doctor.

In some men who have PD, fluid leaks into the scrotum causing swelling of the genitals. This is called a scrotal leak. If you get a scrotal leak, your PD must be stopped temporarily until the leak has healed. Although it is embarrassing, it is important to get the problem seen to immediately.

You will need to have haemodialysis while waiting for the leak to heal.

If the problem continues, you may need a small operation to fix the leak.

I am on PD and I've been told I need a hernia operation. Why has this happened?

A hernia occurs when a wall of muscle weakens and lets an organ or tissue out from inside the abdomen causing a lump to appear. Hernias can cause difficulties for PD patients.

If you already have a hernia before the PD catheter is put in, it can become more of a problem afterwards. The daily draining of PD fluid into and out of the abdomen can cause the hernia to become bigger (and more painful).

If nothing is done, the bowel can become 'stuck' inside the hernia, thereby blocking the bowel. This will require an emergency operation. If the surgeon notices an existing hernia during an operation to insert a PD catheter, it will be repaired during the same operation to stop it causing problems in the future.

Where should I put the APD machine, and what should I do with the used fluid?

Most APD machines are the size of a video recorder – small enough to fit on a bedside table. It is important to remember you will also need an electric plug socket close to the machine.

The used fluid can be drained in two ways. It can either go straight down the drainage pipe in your bathroom, if this is close enough to your bedroom. Or it can be drained into large drainage bags which can be emptied down the toilet in the morning.

Who will pay for my APD machine?

The hospital renal unit should pay for your APD machine.

Some patients have bought their own machines in the past (sometimes with the help of the Kidney Patients Association). But this can cause problems with issues such as maintenance contracts (usually taken out with the hospital and therefore not covering privately-owned machines). These issues need to be clarified before you commit to buying a machine.

APD machines are now more common than they used to be, so

you should never find yourself in a situation where the machine will not be available on the NHS.

What will happen if I don't do all my exchanges?

If you miss out a dialysis exchange occasionally, you may not notice any effects. But missing dialysis regularly will lead to inadequate dialysis and the symptoms of kidney failure will return. These symptoms are:

- weakness and fatigue
- loss of appetite
- nausea
- swollen ankles
- itching.

It is sometimes difficult to recognise symptoms of inadequate dialysis. You can get used to feeling weak and tired, and many patients describe themselves as 'feeling well' because they become accustomed to weakness and fatigue.

However it is important you do get the right amount of dialysis because over a long period of time, inadequate dialysis can cause other more serious problems and even be fatal.

I work full time, and can't believe I will find time to do CAPD. How will I fit in all my exchanges and continue to work?

There are no 'set' times to carry out the exchanges. However, a four bag regimen 'fits' into a typical day. For example, you can do the first bag before breakfast, the second before lunch, the third before your evening meal, and the fourth before going to bed (leaving the fluid in for the last exchange through the night). It is easy for you to adapt the timing of exchanges to your individual needs. For example, if you work during the day, you could delay the midday exchange, and do two 'quick bags' (say, three hours apart) after you come home. Alternatively, you could find a convenient place at work to do the exchange. The nurses at your renal unit will help you talk to the people at work.

When the people who deliver my supplies talk about my CAPD regimen, they refer to '3 by 1' or '2 by 2'. What does this mean?

This refers to the strength of the CAPD fluid used and is 'shorthand' used by many people who work in dialysis units and support services. The first number refers to the weak bags used and the second number refers to the strong bags used. So, a regimen of '3 by 1' would be three weak bags and one strong bag.

When I first went home from hospital after I'd trained to do my CAPD, I didn't have anywhere set up to do my exchanges. It took me quite a few weeks to get sorted out. Is there anything you could suggest for new patients so they don't have the same problem?

It is important to plan your discharge from hospital after you have been trained to do CAPD. You could enlist family and friends to help you set up what you need before you go home.

There are a number of things you will need in order to do CAPD at home.

  (i) A clean washable surface. You can use a large metal or plastic tray or a cut off piece of melamine or Formica.
 (ii) Somewhere to wash your hands near where you plan to do your exchanges. You will also need paper towels or kitchen paper to dry your hands.
(iii) Somewhere to hang the bag of dialysis fluid while it drains into your abdomen. You can use a coat hook, or a coat hanger or even a hat stand. Whatever you use, make sure there is somewhere for you to sit directly underneath.
 (iv) Somewhere to warm the bag of dialysis fluid before you use it. If the fluid is warmed, it will be more comfortable. However, if you put it in cold, it won't do you any harm. Some hospitals supply a special bag warmer. If your hospital doesn't, you can use a hot water bottle in a cool box or you can rest the bag of fluid on the radiator wrapped in a towel. You may also find the airing

cupboard warms the fluid sufficiently. Never warm the fluid in a microwave oven as this can produce hot spots that can damage the peritoneum. Microwave ovens also damage the plastic that the bags are made from and can caramelise the glucose in the solution.

What happens if the phone or doorbell rings while I'm doing my CAPD exchange?

You should wait until you are at a stage in your bag change when it is safe to answer it (either when you are draining the fluid out, draining it in or when you have finished).

Is it possible to go on holiday while on PD?

Going on holiday when you are on dialysis is not only possible but highly recommended. Holidays are a great way to reinforce the fact that you can still enjoy the good things in life as a kidney patient – and they also provide a welcome break for carers.

However, it takes some planning to make sure your treatment requirements go smoothly while you are away. Leave yourself plenty of time between starting the planning process and the time you would like to be away. Inevitably, more exotic locations often involve more planning and notice. As a general guide, you should allow a minimum of three months to make the necessary arrangements. A shorter amount of notice may be possible, depending on your destination.

Detailed advice for travellers on PD is given on pages 173–175.

Haemodialysis

What does going on haemodialysis mean for me? It just feels like the end of the world.

Haemodialysis means different things to different people. But it need not be the end of your life or of your world. Some individuals can have fulfilled and long lives as haemodialysis patients. Some patients carry on full time jobs, some continue to run their own businesses, others study and a few even have successful pregnancies!

Being a kidney patient will mean you have to make some changes to your lifestyle. There will be some restrictions on diet and fluid intake, the inconvenience of thrice weekly visits to the hospital – as well as some occasional medical, psychological and social problems. On the other hand, you will find people just like you who have adapted to life with dialysis. You may make friends with other patients and staff in the renal unit. Dialysis units can have the best atmosphere of any area in the hospital. You will find that, as you become interested in other people there, they also become interested in you. Some dialysis patients who go on to have transplants even claim to miss their visits to the dialysis unit!

I would like to have a haemodialysis machine at home. How do I go about this and who pays?

Your renal unit will bear the cost not only of the machine, but also of the additional plumbing and machinery needed to make the dialysis machine function in your house.

Not all patients are suitable for home haemodialysis – you need to discuss this with the sister or charge nurse in your unit. It is important you have someone at home who is available to help out with the dialysis sessions. Both you and your helper will need special training in dialysis, and in what to do if things go wrong, before you are allowed to dialyse at home. This training can take a reasonably long time, perhaps a month or two. However, with newer teaching techniques the training period is being reduced all the time.

How does blood get to the dialyser? Is it through 'access'? What is 'access' anyway?

During haemodialysis, your blood is taken from your body, cleaned (dialysed) and returned to your body at a rapid rate. An effective haemodialysis session will involve passing all of the blood from your body through the dialyser between 7–15 times. 'Access' is the word doctors and nurses use to describe how they get access to either your bloodstream (in haemodialysis) or inside your peritoneum (in PD, see page 94).

In haemodialysis there are three main types of access.

(i) **Dialysis catheter (lines)**

These are tubes placed into a large vein in your body (usually in your neck or groin) and used to carry blood to and from you during dialysis. The procedure is usually carried out on the ward, where you will be given a local anaesthetic. These lines can be temporary (used for a few weeks) or semi permanent (used for up to one year).

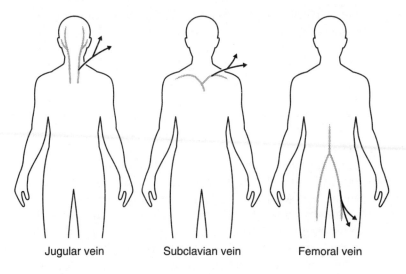

Jugular vein   Subclavian vein   Femoral vein

Figure 9 Entry positions for haemodialysis catheter lines

(ii) **Fistula**

A fistula is formed when an artery is joined to a vein, during an operation. The blood that flows through an artery travels at a much higher pressure than that through a vein. When the blood is diverted from the artery into the vein it causes the vein to enlarge. This enlarged vein

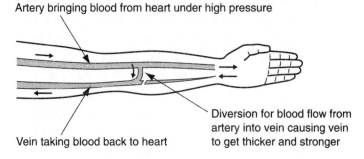

Artery bringing blood from heart under high pressure

Diversion for blood flow from artery into vein causing vein to get thicker and stronger

Vein taking blood back to heart

Figure 10 Position of a fistula

has a 'thrill' or 'bruit' when touched or listened to through a stethoscope because of the rapid blood flow. You can feel the bruit as a buzzing sensation if you place your hand over your fistula. Or you can hear it as a whooshing noise, which might keep you awake at night when you first have the fistula formed. They take 6–8 weeks to develop (grow) into something that can be used for haemodialysis.

(iii) **Graft**

A graft is a small tube, about one centimetre wide. It is made from a synthetic material similar to the non-stick material used to line frying pans. Grafts are used in people with weak veins, which aren't strong enough for a fistula to be created. They may also be used if a fistula has stopped working. Grafts are placed between an artery and a vein, in the arm or leg, during an operation. They carry quite a lot of blood, making them ideal for dialysis. Grafts can be used earlier than fistulae (say after two weeks). In emergencies they can be used straight away.

Needles are inserted into the fistula or graft, to take blood away and return blood to you during dialysis. Your fistula, graft or catheter can be seen as your 'lifeline'. It should not be used for anything other than dialysis, even taking blood for tests.

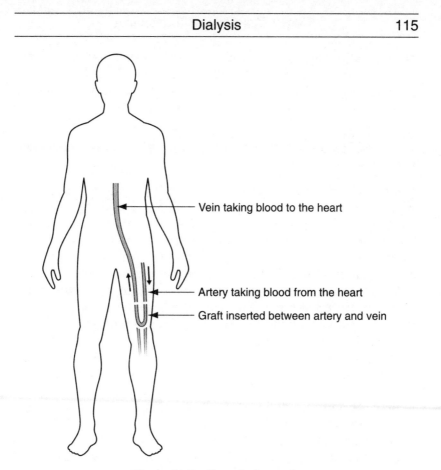

Figure 11 Position of a leg graft

I'm having a fistula put in tomorrow. How soon will I have full use of my arm again?

A fistula is formed by joining an artery to a vein. If the operation is a success, your fistula should buzz or thrill immediately (doctors call this a bruit). Immediately after the operation your arm may be quite painful, bruised and possibly a little swollen. These effects should get better within a few days or weeks. Once your arm has healed, you will be able to use it normally within a couple of weeks. But you will be advised to avoid contact sports and heavy lifting. You should also avoid wearing tight fitting clothes on the arm where your fistula is as this may reduce the flow of blood. Your fistula should be checked at least two or three times a day for the buzz. If this stops, you should contact the hospital immediately.

I'm about to have a fistula operation. What is the success rate like?

Not great, sorry. One problem is that kidney patients often have weak blood vessels, which makes the operation difficult for the surgeon. If you have a brachial (elbow) fistula, there is a 90% chance the operation will be successful, compared to only 60% for radial (wrist) fistulae. These success rates are not great. They are even lower for frail elderly people with weak veins.

Why then do doctors normally try the radial fistula first? It is because, if they do work, they have advantages. They are less likely to 'blow' (bleed into the skin) during a dialysis session. They are less likely to cause a 'steal syndrome' (where the hand goes cold, due to lack of blood). And there is more space (your whole forearm) in which to insert the needles. But many surgeons would rather try a brachial fistula first in a frail elderly patient, or one with diabetes, as for these patients a radial fistula is unlikely to be successful.

You may leave hospital with a fistula that 'works' (ie, you can hear a buzz from it). But this does not necessarily mean it will become a 'good one' – ie, one that can be used time and time again, without any problems. Unfortunately some never become strong enough to use despite working at the start.

If I've had a radial fistula and it does not work, can a brachial fistula be attempted?

If a radial fistula is attempted first but fails, a brachial fistula may still be possible. This is not the case the other way round, however, which is another reason why doctors prefer to try the radial fistula first.

Do fistulas ever stop working?

Yes, it is possible your fistula will stop working. As a general rule, older people and those with diabetes might have problems with their fistulae. Sometimes the blood in your fistula may clot. This can happen if the blood supply through the fistula is restricted.

Caring for your fistula is important – keep it clean and moisturised. Putting the needles into a different spot at each dialysis session may prevent the fistula from growing too big and ugly.

I am on haemodialysis, and have a temperamental fistula. I have been given aspirin. Why is this?

Aspirin is given to thin the blood and stop it from clotting. If the blood clots, it can block a dialysis line or even your fistula. Aspirin is usually taken once a day in the morning. It may irritate the stomach or cause indigestion, but this can be reduced by taking the tablets after food. There are other reasons for being given aspirin – to prevent a heart attack or stroke, for example. Many people take aspirin as a painkiller.

You could also be given an alternative drug called warfarin. This also thins the blood and may prevent fistulae from clotting.

Is a 'dialyser' the same as an 'artifical kidney'? How does it work?

Yes, these are two terms for the same thing.

Dialysers are like short pipes stuffed full of very thin straws. Your blood is taken out of your body via the access (see above), through the machine and through the inside of the 'straws', or hollow fibres. The outside of the hollow fibres are bathed in a constant stream of dialysis fluid. This fluid removes the wastes from the blood.

There are other dialysers, called flat plate dialysers. These use the same principle but the blood flows between sheets of plastic with the dialysis fluid flowing on the outside.

What is in the dialysis fluid?

Dialysis fluid, or dialysate, consists mainly of water. The water used in dialysis fluid is highly purified. That is because your blood will be put in contact with about a pint of water every minute during dialysis. That's about 240 pints during a four hour dialysis session! Dialysis fluid does not contain any of the things you are trying to remove from your blood. Therefore it contains no urea or creatinine. It does contain some of the things your body needs, such as bicarbonate and calcium.

What does the dialysis machine do?

The dialysis machine does many jobs.

(i) It pumps blood from you, via your access, around the machine and back to you.
(ii) It mixes and warms the dialysis fluid which passes through the artificial kidney.
(iii) It monitors what is in the dialysis fluid to make sure the right amounts of the right substances are there throughout the dialysis session.
(iv) It checks the blood for air so that none gets into your bloodstream. Even a small amount of air in your blood can be dangerous.
(v) It monitors the pressure of your blood in your access.

What is a haemodialysis session like? Does it hurt?

When you get to the dialysis unit you will be weighed, and have your blood pressure, pulse rate and temperature recorded. Your weight is important in helping estimate how much fluid you need removing during dialysis. The machine will be fitted with the plastic tubes and dialyser that carry your blood around it. The dialysis fluid will also be set up in the machine. After this you will either sit in a chair or lie on a bed, and the nurse caring for you will clean your access (fistula, graft or line) ready for dialysis and place the needles into your fistula or graft. If you have a catheter,

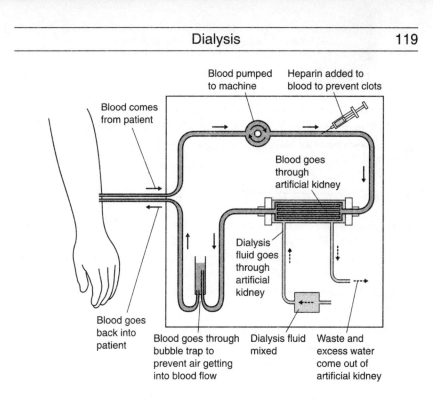

Figure 12 How a haemodialysis machine works

this is attached to the tubes on the machine with screw-in connectors. You will be attached to the machine for the time of your dialysis (usually about three to five hours). In most units you will be given a drink during your time on dialysis, and in some you will also get food.

When your dialysis time is over, the blood in the plastic tubes is 'washed back' into your body using saline (salt water). If you have a fistula or graft, the dialysis needles will then be removed. If you have a line, this will be flushed with saline and the ends filled with heparin (anti-clotting solution). Your blood pressure, pulse rate, temperature and weight will be re-checked to ensure you are safe to go home. If you need an injection of erythropoietin (EPO – see page 52), this will usually be given now.

Haemodialysis usually doesn't hurt. However, some people find that putting the needles into their fistula or graft does hurt. Some also get leg cramps during dialysis, which can be very painful.

Others may lose too much water during a dialysis session, which can lead to very low blood pressure and is called 'going flat'. If this happens, you may feel dizzy, sick, tired and you might vomit and pass out. If you do go flat during dialysis, you will be given some saline through the machine, which quickly helps you to recover.

How often and for how long must I dialyse?

Most people dialyse for between three and five hours, two or three times a week. The length of time depends on how much waste is in your blood, and how big you are. The amount of waste (creatinine and urea) you produce depends on the amount of muscle that you have, as well as the amount of protein in your diet.

My doctor has told me I am 'under dialysing' and he will have to alter my haemodialysis regimen. What is 'under dialysis' and how will he alter my regimen?

The term 'under dialysis' is used when not enough of the waste or extra water is being cleared from your body to keep you healthy, and free from the symptoms of kidney failure.

Waste and extra water are removed by a combination of dialysis and urine (ie what is left of your own kidney function). Almost all patients still have some function of their kidneys remaining when they start dialysis. However, this may decrease with time to the point where no urine at all is produced by the kidneys. It is important to tell the doctor or nurses in the renal unit when you notice you are passing less urine.

When your own kidney function tails off, often shown when you stop passing any urine, it will be necessary to increase the amount of dialysis (or the 'dialysis dose') you receive. Haemodialysis dose can be increased by:

  (i) spending longer on the dialysis machine
 (ii) increasing the speed at which the blood flows through the dialysis machine
(iii) using a bigger or more efficient artificial kidney.

What medicines will I need to take while I'm on haemodialysis?

When you are actually having haemodialysis, you don't usually have to take any medication. Some patients are given a small amount of a liquid version of iron through the dialysis machine. This is given to help EPO work better (see page 52).

There are some other medicines you will have to take regularly whether you are on haemodialysis or PD. These are likely to include calcium carbonate tablets (eg, Calchichew) to help prevent renal bone disease, and EPO for anaemia. You are also likely to need to take drugs to keep your blood pressure low, and reducing your salt intake may also help.

Why do I have to take water tablets now I am on dialysis?

Even when you start dialysis you may still pass a little urine. It won't be enough to enable you not to have dialysis. But large doses of some water tablets (eg, Frusemide) can make you pass a little extra urine. This will be poor quality urine, containing no extra waste products. But it does contain water, so you will be able to drink a little more. Eventually your body may stop producing urine, and when this happens there is no point in taking water tablets.

Water tablets are best taken in the morning and lunchtime if your doctor wants you to take two doses a day. Taking water tablets later in the day may mean you have to get up in the night to go to the toilet. Possible side effects include dizziness, skin rashes with blisters; and gout may also be worsened.

I am on haemodialysis. Can I take cod liver oil capsules for my joints?

It is not a good idea to take cod liver oil capsules when you have kidney failure. They contain lots of Vitamin A, which can build up in your body because your kidneys can't get rid of it. For the same reason, you should not take multivitamin preparations.

What are the long term complications of haemodialysis?

Having haemodialysis for a long time may cause physical problems. Some of these are caused by the disease that caused your kidney failure. Other problems result from the dialysis itself.

(i) **Access problems**

People with diabetes often have problems with haemodialysis access. They may have a fistula formed that doesn't work very well, or even at all. Diabetics also have problems with lines and grafts, as their blood vessels are often thin and fragile. Occasionally, people may use up all of their blood vessels. If this happens, they will have to have PD instead

(ii) **Infections**

Infections are common in people who have haemodialysis. These are often caused by germs, which are brought into the body through the plastic tubes and lines used during dialysis. Unfortunately, people with diabetes are more at risk of getting infections because they are more likely to have to use a line or graft for dialysis.

An infection in your dialysis catheter (or other access) will cause shivering, high temperature and sweating. In very bad cases the infection can spread to other parts of your body and even be life threatening. For example, the infection can spread to your heart.

(iii) **Other problems**

Distressing symptoms such as itching and restless legs are thought to be caused by some of the wastes in the blood. Some men may experience impotence and women of childbearing age may stop having periods.

What about psychological problems? Am I likely to have any of these?

People who have haemodialysis are more prone to depression than the general public. This may be because life on dialysis can seem hopeless to many. Haemodialysis patients may also have a poor self-image, and suffer from physical symptoms such as disturbed sleep, poor appetite, weight loss, constipation and reduced sex drive.

Suicide is considerably more likely among dialysis patients. Anger is also common, and may be caused by problems with having haemodialysis in hospital. There is a lot of waiting time – for treatment, for transport to take you to and from dialysis, for a machine. Angry patients can be uncooperative, deliberately drinking too much or failing to take their medication.

Many haemodialysis patients experience sexual problems and as many as 70% of men on dialysis may be impotent. For more information on psychological or sexual problems, see Chapter 7.

How will I get into hospital for dialysis?

Most hospitals prefer you to use your own transport to get to your dialysis sessions. However, if you have no transport of your own, or you are not well enough to drive, the hospital may be able to provide transport. Haemodialysis is an expensive treatment (costing about £30,000 a year for each patient). It is therefore often only possible to provide transport for patients who have no alternatives.

I'm on haemodialysis, and have smoked since my teens, just as my father and grandfather did. My father is still alive (82 years) and my grandfather lived until he was 90. What are the risks if I carry on smoking?

People with kidney failure have a greater risk of heart disease than the general public. Up to three quarters of those who start haemodialysis show signs of heart damage. Smoking is the biggest single preventable cause of heart disease in the general population. It is best, therefore, to stop smoking as soon as you find out you have kidney failure.

People with kidney failure are more at risk of cancer, and chest infections, than other people. Smoking may increase the risk of both of these. Everyone knows someone who did well despite doing all the 'wrong' things. But we all also know people who did not do well – think about their lifestyle too.

6
Transplants

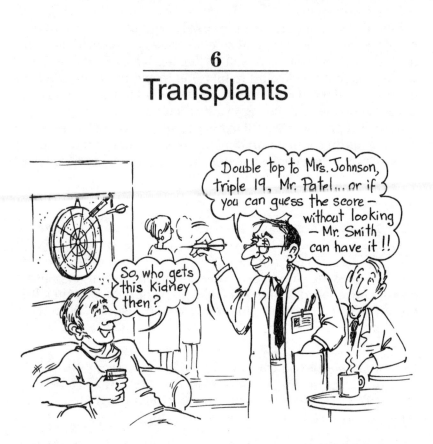

During a kidney transplant operation, a surgeon puts (or transplants) a healthy kidney from someone else (a 'donor') into a patient (or 'recipient'). 'Kidney transplant' is the term used for both the new kidney, and the operation itself.

A successful kidney transplant is the 'best' and most effective treatment for kidney failure. Not everyone is suitable for a transplant however; and not all suitable patients are suitable all the time. Also, before a transplant can take place, it is necessary to find an appropriate donor kidney, which may not be easy.

The first successful kidney transplant operation was performed on 23 December 1954 by Joseph Murray and his team, at the Peter Bent Brigham Hospital, Boston, USA. A kidney was taken from the identical twin brother of a man with kidney failure, and transplanted into the patient. Dr Murray later received a Nobel prize for this work. Today's kidney transplant operation is essentially unchanged, a straightforward operation with a reasonable success rate. Around 85% of kidney transplants are still working at the end of the first year.

After you have had a transplant, you will need to take drugs every day for the rest of your life. If your transplant fails, you can go back to dialysis, and possibly have another transplant.

Availability and suitability

My mother will have to start dialysis in about six months. Can she be put on the transplant waiting list before starting dialysis?

Most renal units in the UK would not put your mother on the national waiting list for a transplant kidney until she was stable on dialysis. However, there are a few that might. Also, some units would put a person with a failing transplant back on the transplant list and give them a new kidney before they have to go back on to dialysis.

Given that it is possible for people with kidney failure to be given a transplant before they need dialysis, why don't all hospitals do it? The reason is that, as there is such a shortage of donor kidneys, many doctors believe it is better if all patients start waiting for a kidney at an equivalent time point – ie, when they start dialysis. The term 'waiting list' is not strictly accurate as there are other factors involved. An available kidney will not be given to the person who has waited the longest, but to the person most suited to receive it. So not everyone who needs a transplant will be able to have one in time.

If a patient has a friend or relative who can donate a kidney to them, they are much more likely to be able to have a transplant when they need one.

Some renal units are undoubtedly organised better in terms of transplantation than others. Some also make more effort to obtain kidneys, and some are 'keener' and work harder to organise living transplants. Find out your unit's position on the National League Table, published every year by an organisation called UK Transplant Support Service Authority.

I have been told I will have to wait at least two years for a kidney transplant. Will it really be this long, and where do the kidneys come from?

In the UK today most kidney transplants are performed using kidneys from cadaveric (dead) donors. Two years is the average waiting time for a cadaveric transplant, but this varies widely. It could be two hours, or 20 years.

Cadaveric donors are people who have been declared brain stem dead in hospital intensive care units. Brain stem death means the donor is completely dead, with no chance of recovery. However, in this situation many organs (including the kidneys) continue to work. The most common cause of death in these people is a head injury resulting from a road traffic accident (99%), or a brain haemorrhage.

In recent years there has been extensive promotion of organ donor cards. Despite this, the number of cadaveric donor kidneys for transplantation still falls short of demand, and is falling every year. There are approximately 1,700 cadaveric kidneys used for transplants in the UK each year. But well over 5,000 people with ESRF are waiting for a transplant. This figure is growing steadily every year.

There are three main reasons why the supply of kidneys does not meet the demand.

  (i) Fewer people are dying in road traffic accidents because of improved health and safety procedures (such as seat belt laws) and improved medical treatments. Therefore, the

number of cadaveric kidneys available for transplants is
falling.

(ii) More people are having dialysis treatment for ESRF, so
there are more who could benefit from a kidney transplant.

(iii) Very few hospitals have a transplant co-ordinator or
adequate facilities. This may mean that potential donors
are missed. (More information about resource issues and
getting involved is given in Chapter 9.)

The National Transplant Waiting List is specifically for
cadaveric transplants (a transplant using a kidney from someone
who has died). About 80–90% of the transplant kidneys in the UK
are from this source. The rest come from living donors known as
'living related transplants' (LRTs), or 'living unrelated transplants'
(LURTs). Other countries where cadaveric organ donation is low
rely heavily on living donors for their kidney transplant
programme. For example, in Norway nearly 50% of the kidneys
transplanted are from live donors – and far more effort is made to
organise living donors than is the case in the UK.

For most patients, the possibility of a transplant kidney from a
living donor will be the best chance of having a transplant
operation before dialysis is needed.

So, why are there so few live transplants done in this country?

For many years it was thought there would be enough cadaveric
kidneys available for everyone on the transplant waiting list.
However, despite many advertising campaigns, this is clearly not
the case.

As a result, live transplants are becoming more common in the
UK, but there is still a large shortfall in the number of kidneys
available. Hopefully, with better awareness of the higher success
rate of live transplants, the number will continue to rise.

While live transplants may seem an obvious solution, there are
a number of personal implications that have to be faced by those
involved.

I am on PD and have recently been diagnosed with breast cancer. What do you think my chances of a kidney transplant are now? And is there an age limit?

Breast cancer is very common, affecting up to 10% of women. It can affect men too, though not as often. So, whether you have kidney failure or not, there is a reasonable chance of getting breast cancer. Some women on dialysis will have both diseases.

Only about 30–40% of patients with kidney failure are suitable for a transplant, provided a suitable donor kidney can be found. You will probably not be considered suitable if you have serious heart disease, have had a major stroke, or have HIV (the virus that causes AIDS) in your blood. If you have a serious type of cancer, like breast cancer, most units would not consider you for a transplant until you have lived five or more years clear of the cancer.

Most renal units do not have an age limit for kidney transplantation. Your suitability for a transplant is assessed on the basis of your general health. Having said that, most kidney doctors would think seriously before transplanting a person over the age of 70. This is because older patients often do not tolerate the transplant operation very well. Also, the drugs needed after a transplant are often too strong for them.

What happens to the kidneys of people who die without donor cards?

Just because someone carries a donor card, this does not automatically mean their organs will be used for transplantation. When a person dies, their body becomes the property of the State. However, their organs cannot be removed for transplantation without the consent of their next of kin.

If someone dies without having a donor card, their next of kin may still be asked for permission to use their organs. But it will be easier for doctors to broach the subject of organ donation with the relatives if the dead person has made their intentions clear. So it is important to carry a donor card if you wish your organs to be used after your death.

Am I equally likely to get a kidney transplant in all UK renal units, or is there a 'postcode lottery'?

Some renal units make more of an effort to obtain cadaveric organs than others. As most people have two kidneys, the surgeon who removes the kidneys from the cadaveric donor will usually send one away to another renal unit in the UK where it is given to the best-matched patient. The other kidney is kept for the best-matched patient locally. Therefore, units that remove more organs will transplant more patients.

This system is beginning to change for the better, but ask your transplant surgeon what the record is like in your area.

Are rich and famous people more likely to get a kidney transplant quicker than I am?

No. The rich and famous are no more likely to get kidneys than 'ordinary' people. It is also illegal to buy a kidney in the UK.

Why can't doctors transplant a kidney from anyone into me?

For a kidney transplant to be successful, it is essential that the tissues of the new kidney are fairly similar to yours – what doctors call 'a good match'. A kidney that is not a good match is more likely to cause your body's natural defence system to attack and 'reject' it from your body (see page 143).

Before a suitable kidney can be found, you need to have a number of tests. The most important of these are to find out your blood group and tissue type. The results will then be checked against the results of similar tests carried out on the donor.

I'm blood group 'O'. What does this mean?

Your blood group is an inherited characteristic of the red blood cells in your body and stays the same throughout your life. There are four main blood groups: A, B, AB and O. Group O is the most common (55%), group A is the second most common (35%).

Your blood group depends on whether or not you have certain substances called antigens (types of protein) in your body. Two different antigens – called A and B – determine a person's blood group. If you have these antigens, they will be on the outer surface of all your cells, not just on your blood cells. If you have only antigen A, your blood group is A. If you have only antigen B, your blood group is B. If you have both antigen A and antigen B, your blood group is AB. If you have neither of these antigens, your blood group is O.

For a kidney transplant to work, must the donor and recipient have the same blood group?

Blood group matching is essential, even though the function of the blood group antigens is not clear. In practice, the blood group seems to act as a 'friendly face' for your cells – so the rest of the body can recognise the cells as your own, and not fight them off. Your immune system will attack any cells that have different antigens to your own. You can only be given a transplant kidney if your blood group and that of the donor are matched as follows.

You	Donor
Group O	Group O
Group A	Group A or group O
Group B	Group B or group O
Group AB	Any group (O, A, B, or AB)

So as you can see, people who have blood group O can only have an O kidney, whereas people with blood group AB can have a kidney from anyone. Also, O kidneys can be given to any patient.

This is the same for both cadaveric and living transplants.

The doctor has done a blood test to assess my 'tissue type'. What does this mean?

The tissue type is another set of antigens (proteins which live on the surface of most of your cells) that we try to match. Unlike blood group matching, tissue type matching is desirable – to improve the chances of the kidney lasting a long time – but not essential. As with blood matching, you and the donor kidney are matched using a blood test. The tissue typing test shows your genetic make-up (sometimes called your 'genetic fingerprint').

Your tissue type is something you are born with and stays the same throughout your life. The cells are the tiny microscopic building blocks of your body. You have only one tissue type, just as you only have one blood group, but your tissue type is made up of many different tissue type proteins. However, we look at the six proteins that we feel are the most important ones, and we say that these are your tissue type (in fact, they are only part of it).

The three main tissue type proteins we choose are called A, B and DR. Everyone has two of each, making six in all. There are many different versions of each A, B and DR. This means there are hundreds of different possible tissue type combinations. For example, your tissue type could be A1/A2, B7/B8, DR2/DR3.

Because there are so many possible tissue types, perfectly matching your tissue type is more complicated than matching your blood group. Basically, the more tissue type proteins that are the same for you and your donor kidney, the better the chances are that the transplant kidney will work.

Given the large number of tissue type possibilities, it is unusual (15% of cases in the UK) to get an exact match between you and the donor. This called a '6 out of 6 match', or a 'full-house match'. The only people who will definitely be a 6 out of 6 match are identical twins. Siblings (brothers and sisters) have a one in four chance of being a 6 out of 6 match. Most renal units will offer a you a transplant if you and the donor have three or more of the six tissue type characteristics in common.

For example, a transplant might be offered in the following situation:

| **You:** | **A1**/A2 | **B7**/B8 | **DR2**/DR3 |
| **Donor:** | **A1**/A3 | **B7**/B12 | **DR2**/DR7 |

As the A1, B7 and DR2 proteins are the same in this example, it would be called a '3 out of 6 match'.

The more proteins that match, the longer the kidney is likely to work. So a '6 out of 6 match' is better than a '3 out of 6 match'. The better the match, the more likely that your body will accept the kidney 'as your own', and not try to reject it. Unfortunately, there is no guarantee your body will not reject the best possible match, a '6 out of 6' match. This is because the blood group and tissue type are not the only cell surface proteins that are important on your cells. Doctors have not yet been able to find these other important proteins.

Which is more important, the tissue type or the blood group match?

The blood group is much more important than the tissue type. So it is essential to have a kidney with a matched blood group, but the tissue type match does not have to be perfect. In fact if you are having a living transplant, the blood group is the only match that really matters.

I am Asian and on PD. I've been told I will have to wait longer than a white person for a kidney transplant. Is my renal unit being racist?

In the UK, organs are distributed mainly according to blood group and tissue type. Unfortunately, this means that Asian patients often have to wait longer for a transplant than other patients. This is not due to racism, but because Asian people have different blood groups and tissue types from white people. As most cadaveric kidney donors are white, doctors will be less likely to find a kidney to suit an Asian patient. It is particularly important therefore for Asian relatives, friends and partners to offer a kidney to the patient. This is likely to be much safer too than buying a kidney abroad.

I want to go onto the kidney transplant waiting list, but don't know what is involved. What steps do I go through?

First, you will be tested for blood group and tissue type (see above). After these tests, there are several more stages you have to go through.

Before you can be put forward for a transplant, you will have to be tested for various viruses. These include HIV (the virus that causes AIDS), hepatitis B, hepatitis C and cytomegalovirus (known as CMV). It is important to test for these viruses because they may be dormant ('sleeping', causing no symptoms) in your body. After the transplant, they may be 'woken up' and cause illness.

If you refuse to have any of these tests, you will not be able to have a kidney transplant. Having one of the viruses does not necessarily mean you will not get a transplant, it just means the doctors will have to be more careful. At present, testing positive for HIV does mean you won't be offered a transplant. This is because you won't be able to tolerate the drugs you have to take afterwards. It may change as the treatments for HIV improve.

Other tests necessary before a transplant include an electro-cardiogram (ECG, an electric recording of the heart beat), a chest X-ray and sometimes an echocardiogram (ECHO, a sound-wave picture of the heart). If you have diabetes, some renal units also require you to have a cardiac catheter test (a special X-ray picture of the heart). This is because people with diabetes sometimes have serious heart problems which would affect the chance of the transplant being successful. However, the investigation itself is not without risk.

If you have had problems with the blood vessels in your legs, you may be asked to have a Doppler ultrasound. If this shows bigger problems, it may mean you also need a femoral arteriogram, a special X-ray picture of the leg arteries.

This combination of tests is called a 'transplant work-up'. If all the results are satisfactory, you can then be put on the national waiting list for a cadaveric transplant, or be considered for a possible transplant from a living donor. It is quite likely one or more of these tests will indicate a need for additional, more complex tests.

I'm on haemodialysis and have been on the waiting list for a transplant for five years. I've never been offered one. A chap who dialyses on my shift got a kidney after only two months. This does not seem a very fair waiting list. What is going on?

You have been unlucky. Waiting five years is longer than average, though it is by no means unheard of. The average waiting time for a transplant is about two years. It is important to note this is an average – it can be two hours, or twenty years.

The waiting list works on the basis of finding the 'best' patient for the donor kidney, when one becomes available. In this way, it is not a true waiting list – organised on a first in, first out basis. Transplants are allocated to the patient who is the best match for the kidney in terms of blood group and tissue type. In other words, when you were put on the waiting list five years ago, you did not join a queue, knowing your name will come up after a reasonably fixed time. This is why the chap who dialyses on your shift got a kidney so soon. He was just lucky, as his blood group and tissue type was a better match for that kidney than yours.

Can I be taken off the waiting list? If so, will I be informed?

It may sometimes be necessary to take you off the transplant waiting list, either temporarily or permanently. This may happen, for example, if you develop a serious infection or a heart problem, or if you need a major operation. This decision is not made lightly. If you are removed from the list, you should be told about the decision, and informed whether your removal from the list is temporary or permanent. If you are unsure whether you are 'on the list', you should ask. If you are really concerned, ask to see the evidence that you are still on the list, in writing.

The doctor is not, in fact, legally required to tell you if you have been taken off the list. So it is important you make sure you are still on the list, every time you see your doctor or nurse.

Just because you were once suitable for a kidney transplant, it does not mean you always will be. As you get older, whether you have kidney failure or not, you are more liable to get heart attacks, strokes and cancer. If any of these things happen, you may be taken off the waiting list permanently. This is one of the reasons it is important to have a kidney transplant as soon as possible, if you are suitable. Most importantly, it is best to have a living transplant (from a friend, partner or relative) as soon as it is necessary. Then you do not have to wait at all.

What will happen if a kidney becomes available and the unit cannot find me?

If you are on the waiting list for a transplant, you may not be given much notice when a kidney becomes available. If you cannot be found, the kidney will be offered to someone else, so ensure that the unit has contact numbers for you at all times – in these days of mobile phones and bleepers, there is no excuse for you to be difficult to get hold of. Not being contactable on one night could mean you have to wait several more years for the next call.

Tell your unit if you go on holiday. You may not have to come off the list if you are abroad and can return within twelve hours, so don't go too far.

My son is a 23-year-old haemodialysis patient who has had three failed transplants. He has now been back on dialysis for four years, but has never been offered a kidney. I've been told that one of the reasons is that he has 'high antibodies' making him 'untransplantable'. Why?

Antibodies are proteins made by your lymphocytes (specialist white blood cells). Their normal job is to attack and destroy germs in your blood, and other invaders to your body. The new kidney will stimulate your lymphocytes to make antibodies to reject that kidney. These antibodies never disappear. This leads to two problems. Firstly, if you stop taking your immuno-suppressant drugs, the antibodies can become active, and reject the kidney. Secondly, if the kidney fails, and you have another kidney, the antibodies may try to reject the new kidney.

Some patients develop lots of antibodies, especially if they have had two or more failed transplants. While the term 'untransplantable' is not strictly accurate and can be very discouraging, it is true to say a further transplant will be unlikely to work unless the antibodies can be cleared.

A technique called immuno-adsorption can sometimes help 'untransplantable' patients such as your son not to reject another kidney. Unfortunately, it is not available in most renal units, partly because the success rate is not great (around 50%) and partly because it is very expensive.

The operation and after

What are the pros and cons of having a kidney transplant?

For some people a successful kidney transplant can give the best quality of life, of all the available treatments. There is no doubt that for the right person at the right time, it is the best treatment option. A 'good' transplant provides about 50% of the function of two normal kidneys (compared with only about 5% from either type of dialysis).

The most obvious advantage of a successful transplant is freedom from dialysis. Also, there are no particular fluid or dietary restrictions after a transplant, and you can stop some of the tablets and injections you were taking while on dialysis (eg, Calcichew and EPO). Most people who have had a transplant often feel better and have more energy than they did on dialysis. They find it easier to work and their sex life improves.

As with any major procedure, there are risks associated with a kidney transplant.

- **The transplant kidney may not work**
  About 15% of transplant kidneys are not working at the end of the first year. This is sometimes due to 'rejection', ie your body recognises that the transplanted kidney is not 'its own' and tries to 'reject' it from the body (see page 143).

- **Drug side effects**
  After a kidney transplant, you need to take several strong

drugs every day. These help to prevent rejection but have serious side effects (see pages 163–170).

- **Cancer**
  The most serious side effect of the drugs you have to take is a type of cancer called lymphoma. This can kill you.

About 5% of people who have a kidney transplant will die within one year of the operation. However, it is perfectly possible they would have died within that time if they had stayed on dialysis, depending on their general health. Even allowing for these risks, most doctors believe a kidney transplant to be the best treatment for many patients most of the time.

What will happen when I'm called up for a transplant?

Don't panic. Make your way to the hospital soon, but there is no need to rush. Having said that, it is worth thinking in advance about how you might get to hospital if the call comes through at 4 am – keeping a reasonable amount of petrol in your car for example, or having numbers for all night taxi services by the phone.

If you are called up to go into hospital for a transplant, you are not guaranteed to receive it. Before the operation can go ahead, it is necessary to check you are well enough for major surgery, and will not reject the transplant kidney immediately after the operation. When you arrive at the hospital you will undergo the following tests.

(i) **Physical examination**
  A doctor will give you a thorough physical examination, to check it is safe to proceed. For example, if you have a heavy cold, it may considered too risky for you to have an anaesthetic. If you are not fit enough, you will be sent home and put back on the waiting list.

(ii) **The cross-match**
  This test is the final hurdle and is different to a tissue type or blood group match. The cross match is a blood test to check you have no antibodies (substances that normally help the body to fight infection) that would react with the donor kidney. High levels of such antibodies in the blood

mean the new kidney is likely to be rejected as soon as it is put into you, even if it seems a good tissue type match.

A cross-match is done by mixing a sample of your blood with cells from the donor's body. These cells come from donor's lymph glands or spleen. If your blood does not start attacking the donor's cells, it is assumed you will be less likely to reject the new kidney. This is called a negative cross-match, and means the operation can go ahead. So, a negative cross-match is good.

If the cross-match is positive (ie, your blood reacts to the donor's cells), you will be sent home and put back on the waiting list. This can be disappointing, but it is much better to return to dialysis for a while than be given a kidney that doesn't work and may make you extremely ill.

What does the operation actually involve? Will my old kidneys be taken out?

First you will be put to sleep with a general anaesthetic. The operation lasts two to three hours. The surgeon makes a diagonal cut into the abdomen, to one side below the navel.

Your own kidneys are usually left in place. The transplant kidney is placed lower in the abdomen, just above your groin. The transplant kidney has its own artery (to take blood to it), vein (to take blood from it) and ureter (to take urine to the bladder).

The artery belonging to the new kidney is attached to the main artery supplying blood to your leg on that side of the body. The vein belonging to the new kidney is attached to the main vein carrying blood from that leg. These leg blood vessels are big enough to send blood to and from the new kidney without affecting the blood supply to your leg. Problems with the vein can lead to leg swelling (on the side of the transplant) after the operation. This is usually temporary. The transplant kidney's ureter is attached to your own bladder.

A small plastic tube (a 'double J stent') is usually inserted into the ureter to help prevent it from becoming blocked after the operation. At the end of the operation, your abdomen is closed with stitches.

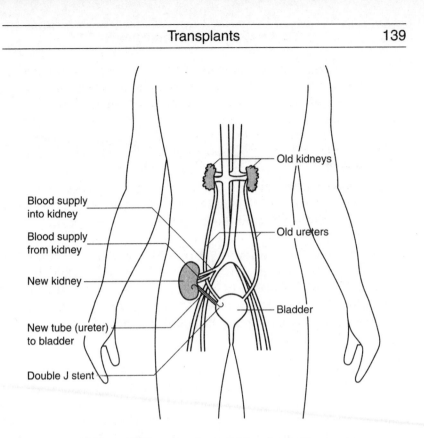

Figure 13 The transplanted kidney in position

What happens immediately after the operation? Will I be in intensive care?

When you wake up from the anaesthetic, you are likely to be back on your ward, or (in some hospitals) in a high dependency ward for the first day or two. So you shouldn't be in the intensive care unit.

You will have several tubes coming out of your body. These may include the following.

    (i) A urinary catheter (a tube which takes urine out of your bladder).

(ii) A central venous pressure (CVP) line, which is placed under your collarbone or in the side of your neck. The CVP line measures the pressure of blood inside your heart.

(iii) An intravenous drip in your arm. This will be used to give you fluid and drugs you might need.

(iv) One or more surgical drains coming out of your abdomen. The drain will help to drain off any excess fluid that gathers around the kidney after the operation.

These tubes will be removed one by one over the next few days. The urinary catheter is usually left in place for five days or more. This is because your bladder may not be used to storing the large amounts of urine your new kidney may be producing. The urinary catheter also enables accurate measurement of the amount of urine passed.

The double J stent (see above) is usually removed during a small operation (under either a local or general anaesthetic) about three months after the transplant. PD patients will usually have their catheter left in for a while. Some haemodialysis patients find their fistula stops working at some stage after the transplant. This does not matter, because if the transplant is working well, you will not need it.

The first few days after the operation are critical and you will be monitored closely. Particular attention is paid to your blood pressure, fluid intake and urine output. Most patients are able to drink and eat small amounts, and sit out of bed on the day after the operation.

You will have your blood creatinine level (see pages 28–29) measured every day. This shows whether or not the transplant kidney is working. The amount of urine the new kidney makes is not a reliable indicator, as you may produce a large volume of urine that does not contain many toxins.

In about one third of kidney transplants, the kidney does not produce any urine in the first few days or sometimes weeks after the transplant. This does not mean the transplant will never work. However, transplants that work from the start are more likely to last a long time. If the transplant does not work straightaway, you will need to continue dialysis until it does. A 'good transplant' is one that is working well after one year, not after two weeks. Ideally, the blood creatinine level should fall to below about 150 micromoles per litre and stay at this level.

How long will I be in hospital?

Most people stay in hospital for about two weeks after the operation.

How often will I have to come back to the hospital after I leave?

After leaving hospital, you will need to go to clinic frequently for many months. At first you will have to go to hospital two or three times per week, then once a week, then once every two weeks. When the doctors are satisfied your kidney is working well, your appointments may be reduced to once every three months or so. This is not usually until after the first year, if everything is stable.

How long will I have to take off work after a transplant?

It usually takes three to six months for you to return to normal activities, including work. It is recommended you do not drive for at least one month after a transplant operation.

We suggest you plan to have three months off work, but tell the bosses that 6–12 months could be necessary.

How long after my transplant operation will my partner and I have to wait before having sex again?

Neither the function of the kidney, nor the risk of infection, will be affected by having sex. But it is probably better to wait around four weeks after leaving hospital before resuming sexual activity.

How long will the transplanted kidney last?

A kidney transplant does not last forever. The average life-span of a transplanted kidney is eight years for a cadaveric kidney, and eleven years for a living related transplant. The average for a living unrelated transplant is somewhere between the two. So, the 'best' (longest lasting) kidney transplant is one from a relative, then a friend or partner, then a dead person.

Another way of estimating how long a transplanted kidney will last is to look at the percentage chance it has of being effective at set time points. A transplanted cadaveric kidney has, on average:

(i) an 85% chance of working one year after the operation;

(ii) a 60% chance of lasting five years;

(iii) a 50% chance of lasting ten years or more.

The chances that a kidney donated by a living person will be working at these time points are about 10% better.

If you are young when you have your first transplant, whatever type it is, you may need two or more transplants in your life.

Are there any general guidelines to help me keep my kidney working?

There are things you can do to help yourself. You should always:

(i) take the immunosuppressant drugs as prescribed;

(ii) attend appointments as requested;

(iii) seek advice from the renal unit as soon as a problem is experienced.

What happens if my transplant doesn't work?

If your transplant fails, you can go back on dialysis. You may also be able to have another transplant. You may have to wait six months or so, either to be put back on the transplant waiting list or have a kidney from a friend or relative. It can take that long too for the body to become strong enough for another operation. Before you can be put back on the transplant waiting list, you will have to go through the transplant work-up process again. When you have your first transplant, you are obviously considered fit enough for it. But when the transplant fails, your general health may deteriorate and you may no longer be suitable for such a major procedure. A doctor's decision not to offer you another transplant is a difficult one, which would not be made lightly. But if you are not happy with the decision, you could always ask for a second opinion from a kidney doctor in another unit.

What is rejection and how is it treated?

'Rejection' means your body recognises that the transplanted kidney is not its own and tries to reject it from your body. Even when you and the transplant kidney are apparently well-matched in terms of blood group and tissue type, some degree of rejection is common.

The body system responsible for the rejection process is called the immune system. This is the body's natural defence system and is located all over the body. It includes organs such as the bone marrow, spleen and appendix, lymph nodes including the glands in the neck, and specialist white blood cells called lymphocytes.

The task of the immune system is to fight foreign invaders. These include germs (such as bacteria and viruses) and foreign objects (such as splinters or thorns embedded in the skin). The immune system also fights cancer. An individual's immune system does not usually attack that person's own cells because these all have a 'friendly face' consisting of special proteins called antigens on the outer surface of the cells. The immune system recognises the friendly face and knows to leave the cells alone. Germs and foreign objects do not have this friendly face. Nor do cancer cells, which have developed in an abnormal way.

Normally, the immune system is a good thing, protecting the body from dangerous infections, foreign bodies and cancer. But after a transplant it can be a bad thing. If the immune system recognises that the new kidney does not have the usual friendly face of the body's own cells, it will become overactive and send lymphocytes to attack and reject the kidney. The body is actually trying to protect you from the kidney, which it perceives as a danger. Luckily, there are drugs – **immunosuppressants** – that can help prevent and treat the rejection process.

There are two types of rejection. If rejection occurs early after a transplant, it is called **acute rejection**. If it occurs after the first couple of years, it is more likely to be **chronic rejection**.

What is acute rejection?

Acute rejection is short-term, of rapid onset, and requires immediate action. It usually occurs in the first few weeks or months after a transplant. It is very common – about 40% of patients will experience acute rejection in the first three months following a transplant. Good matching of tissue type reduces the risk of acute rejection. If it hasn't occurred within one year of the operation, it is unlikely to happen. But if you were to stop taking your immunosuppressant tablets, acute rejection will occur no matter how long you have had the kidney.

The severity of acute rejection is variable. Severe rejection is rare, but when it occurs it can lead to loss of the kidney. Moderate or mild rejection is more common and is relatively easy to reverse.

Acute rejection may sometimes cause pain and fever, but usually there are no obvious symptoms. Doctors will suspect you have acute rejection if the blood creatinine either fails to come down after a transplant, or if it starts to fall then remains stable or increases again. However, acute rejection is not the only reason for problems with blood creatinine levels after a transplant, and these other possibilities will be explored too.

How will the doctors know if my kidney has acute rejection?

The only way to be sure whether a transplant kidney is being rejected is to do a **biopsy**. This test involves the removal of a very small piece of the new kidney, which is then examined under a microscope for signs of rejection. It is common to have two or more biopsies in the weeks after the operation.

This procedure does carry small risks:

(i) a 1 in 20 chance of not getting sufficient tissue (it will then need to be repeated the next day);

(ii) a 1 in 100 chance of a small bleed from the kidney;

(iii) a 1 in 1000 chance of the bleeding being so bad that the kidney will have to be removed, so you will need to go back on dialysis;

(iv) a 1 in 10,000 chance of dying.

Your doctor will do everything possible to make the biopsy safe.

How is acute rejection treated?

If the biopsy shows signs of rejection, you will be given a high-dose of a steroid drug, either prednisolone or methyl-prednisolone. This will be given by tablet (prednisolone), or intravenous injection (methylprednisolone), once a day for three days. These are called 'pulses'. Usually, this treatment will slow down or even stop the rejection process, and the creatinine level in the blood will start to decrease.

If the first course of three pulses of steroid do not work, some doctors might give you another course. Alternatively, you may be given a 5–10 day course of a stronger intravenous injection, such as anti-lymphocyte globulin (ALG), anti-thymocyte globulin (ATG) or orthoclone K T-cell receptor 3 (OKT3) antibody. These almost always work and the rejection process goes away. However, all of them can have unpleasant side effects, especially OKT3 which can cause fever, diarrhoea, joint and muscle pain, wheezing, and shortness of breath due to fluid on the lungs (pulmonary oedema).

Another option is to change your cyclosporin, if you are on it, to an alternative slightly stronger drug called tacrolimus (though some units start all the patients off on tacrolimus). Your azathioprine (if you are on it) can be changed for a newer slightly stronger drug called mycophenolate.

What is chronic rejection and how is it different to acute rejection?

Chronic rejection may take years to happen, but it is the most common cause of transplant failure after the first year. It is very different from acute rejection. Your immune system does not attack and reject the transplant kidney – chronic rejection is more like a slow ageing of the new kidney.

The cause of chronic rejection is uncertain. Doctors may suspect chronic rejection if your blood creatinine starts to rise slowly after it has been stable for some time. As with acute rejection, the only sure way to diagnose the condition is by biopsy. However, as there is no treatment for chronic rejection, some doctors prefer to avoid this.

The severity of chronic rejection varies. Mild chronic rejection is not usually a problem, but a more severe form will eventually lead to failure of the kidney and the need to restart dialysis or have another transplant.

Apart from rejection, what other complications might I get after a transplant?

Infection is a major complication. The immunosuppressant drugs you take help prevent transplant rejection by making your immune system less efficient. Therefore, they also reduce your ability to fight infections. There is no guaranteed way of avoiding infection, though it is a good idea to keep away from people who have infections, especially babies and young children.

While most people taking immunosuppressant drugs manage to avoid too many problems, there is one infection that is particularly hazardous for transplant patients. This is called cyto-megalovirus (CMV). For people with healthy immune systems, CMV is a mild infection that causes a 'flu-like illness. However, if you have just received a transplant, CMV infection can be severe. The treatment for CMV is a drug called gancyclovir, which is given as a course of injections.

The immune system attacks foreign invaders that enter the body. It also fights off cancer that occurs inside the body. To stop a kidney transplant being rejected, immunosuppressant drugs have to be taken every day. Not surprisingly, a suppressed and weakened immune system is less able to fight off cancer, so you are more likely to get cancer after you have had a transplant.

If I have a transplant, how much more likely am I to get cancer than other people? And what type of cancer should I look out for?

Overall, if you have a kidney transplant you will be about four times more likely to get cancer of some type. If you have had a transplant for a long time, such as 25 years, you have around a 70% chance of suffering some type of cancer. But this figure does include skin cancers which are not normally life-threatening.

You will have a much greater risk of getting a skin cancer. If you live in a country with a lot of sunshine the risk is higher – for example, in Australia, it is 21 times higher. If you live in a murky country like the UK, the risk is up to seven times greater.

Skin cancer will not normally kill you. You may need frequent and sometimes substantial surgery to keep it at bay. It is important that all transplant patients look after their skin. You should protect yourself from the sun (how to do this is described in more detail in the travel section, on pages 172–184). It is also important to keep a close eye on all of your skin all the time, and report any suspicious lumps that appear (especially ones that enlarge, or change colour) to your doctor immediately.

There is another common cancer that affects people who have had a transplant. This is called lymphoma and is a cancer of the immune system. A small number (1–2%) of transplant patients will develop lymphoma, usually within a year of the operation. This cancer affects cells in the body's immune system (mainly in the spleen and lymph nodes), and can be fatal in up to 50% of cases.

Some patients, have a milder form of lymphoma which goes away when the doses of your immunosuppressant drugs are reduced. It may even be necessary to stop the immuno-suppressant drugs altogether, which will mean you might reject (and lose) your transplant kidney and need to start dialysis again.

The symptoms of lymphoma include weight loss, diarrhoea, flu-like symptoms, enlarged glands or lumps in the neck, armpit or groin, a sore throat that doesn't get better, abdominal pain and bleeding from the back passage. Lymphoma may be found by chance at an emergency operation. If you get any of these symptoms, report them to your doctor immediately.

Cancer of the cervix (the 'neck' of the womb) is also more common in women who have had a transplant. They are about 15 times more likely than other women to get the disease. Fortunately, cervical cancer is easy to treat if it is picked up early. So women who have had a transplant should have a cervical smear test every year. This test can pick up abnormalities before they turn into cancer and treatment can be given straight away. Treatments include laser therapy, a 'cone biopsy' (removal of the end of the cervix) or a hysterectomy (removal of the womb).

Is there any chance I might get other forms of cancer such as lung cancer or breast cancer?

You are no more likely to get lung or breast cancer if you have had a transplant than anyone else. However, this does not mean you won't get lung or breast cancer.

There are some rare types of cancer for which transplant patients are at greater risk than other people. These include liver cancer, cancer of the lip, of the vulva (the area around the vagina) and of the anus. Another very rare cancer is Kaposi's sarcoma, a form of skin cancer. This is now most common in patients with AIDS ('Acquired Immunodeficiency Syndrome'), because the virus suppresses patients' immune systems. Kaposi's sarcoma also occurs in transplant patients because the immuno-suppressant drugs (used to prevent rejection) suppress the immune system and put patients into an AIDS-like state.

There is not a lot you can do to prevent these cancers. You should always report any strange lump promptly to your doctor.

Will having a kidney transplant affect my mouth? Should I have regular dental checks?

The new kidney will not itself affect your teeth. But it is necessary to suppress the immune system after transplant, and this makes you susceptible to all infections including those of the gums and teeth. So, after a transplant, it is especially important to keep the mouth clean with regular brushing, flossing and visits to the dental hygienist.

You should make sure your dentist knows you are a kidney patient. Avoid dental checkups for three months after the transplant to let everything settle down. Your dentist needs to be aware that you are taking immunosuppressants as this will affect prescribing of antibiotics before and after any dental procedure. Your dentist may need to write to your kidney consultant for advice before any treatment is given.

I am a diabetic on dialysis. I've heard about a 'double transplant' (kidney and pancreas). Are they done in the UK and do they work?

This is a new operation, first performed in the late 1990s, and is still relatively uncommon. However, many people who have had a double transplant have done well. They no longer need dialysis, nor do they need insulin injections. This may help to slow down some of the other complications of diabetes, such as damage to the eyes.

You should ask your doctor if your renal unit performs this type of operation. If your unit does not do them, and you want to be considered for a double transplant, you will have to ask to be referred to a unit that does. They do perform these transplants on patients from other renal units.

The major disadvantage is that the operation is technically more difficult for the surgeon. In a 'standard' kidney transplant, it is unusual for you to require any further significant operations after the initial surgery. However, after a kidney–pancreas transplant, it is quite common for you to have one or more significant operations in the three months after the operation.

Patients often spend 1–2 months in hospital after a kidney–pancreas transplant, compared to the 'normal' two weeks or so.

You may have to take extra tablets after a kidney–pancreas transplant, in particular, an unpleasant tasting tablet called sodium bicarbonate. If this is necessary, you may be asked to take 12 or more of them every day.

Some units now offer a new type of transplant to diabetic patients, called an **islet cell transplant**. The islet cells are that part of the pancreas that makes insulin. The transplant involves an injection of islet cells from the pancreas into the patient's liver. They 'stick' there, and grow, and start to make insulin. If this type of transplant could be combined with a kidney transplant, it would solve both major problems affecting a patient with diabetes and kidney failure. Research is continuing to see whether such a double treatment is possible and safe. In theory it should be.

I've read about research into animal transplant donors in the papers. Is it possible to take a kidney from a pig and put it into a human?

The term xenotransplantation refers to the possibility of using organs taken from animals (especially pigs) for transplantation into humans. A certain amount of research has been done in this area, but the problems are currently considered too great for this type of transplant to be used. One major concern is the risk of passing on animal viruses to humans.

I've had a transplant and I have changed to a low-tar brand of cigarettes, with a filter. Why is smoking harmful now?

Rejection of your transplant kidney from your body is prevented by the use of immunosuppressant drugs. Unfortunately these drugs also mean the whole body is increasingly susceptible to infection and cancer. Smoking increases the risk of lung cancer as well as cancers of the mouth and throat. It is not just the tar content of cigarettes that is responsible for cancers.

People on immunosuppressant drugs also have an increased risk of heart disease and smoking plays a part in this. Good quality research has recently demonstrated that kidney failure advances quickest in individuals who smoke, especially those with high blood pressure. It is not certain whether this will apply to transplant patients – only you know if this is a risk you are prepared to take.

Other research shows it is not only the tar in cigarette smoke which can damage your health. Tobacco also contains fungal spores, which are responsible for up to 95% of fungal infections in people recovering from a transplant operation.

The safe and simple advice is to stop, although that is not always easy. Seek help from your doctor, nurse or counsellor. Some people find acupuncture or hypnosis helpful (your GP should be able to refer you). Or use patches or gum.

Living transplants

Is a live transplant better than a cadaveric transplant, and if so why?

There are many benefits to having a live transplant.

Accepting a kidney from a loved one means the wait for a transplant may be shorter than for a cadaveric transplant. In some circumstances the transplant may take place before you need to start dialysis. The transplant operation can also be planned in advance, on a date suitable for everyone involved, whereas cadaveric transplants often happen at very short notice.

A kidney from a live donor is likely to function for longer than a cadaveric kidney – on average eleven years compared to eight years.

A kidney from a live donor is usually of better quality than a cadaveric kidney. This is because live donors are carefully screened for any diseases that might affect their kidneys such as hypertension or diabetes. The donor's kidneys are also checked to make sure they function perfectly.

While cadaveric kidneys for transplantation are never of poor quality, they do come from people from a range of ages and there is often no time to determine the exact function of the kidney before use. Also, the donor may have died a traumatic death.

A live transplant may improve the relationship between donor and recipient, as there is a common bond. There is also evidence to suggest the recipient of a live transplant is more likely to take the medication required after the transplant, perhaps because the recipient feels more of a responsibility towards looking after the new kidney.

Does a live donor have to be related to the recipient?

Most live donor transplants are performed using kidneys from people who are related to each other, such as genetically related family members. These are called 'living related transplants' (LRTs).

An increasing number of live kidney transplants use organs from people who are not genetically related, although they do have a 'relationship' with each other. This could be through marriage, co-habitation or a long-standing friendship. Whatever the circumstances, before any live transplant can go ahead, the relationship must be proven.

If donor and recipient are from the same family, the relationship can be proved from blood samples. If the relationship is an emotional one (husband, wife, partner or friend), it must be established in other ways. In these situations each case must be reported to ULTRA (Unrelated Live Transplant Regulatory Authority), an authority established in Law by the Human Organ Transplants Act, 1989. ULTRA's role is to ensure the kidney is being donated freely and for no other reason than to benefit the recipient's health. ULTRA has a panel of members consisting of a medical chairman and two lay members, all of whom will assess the suitability of each application.

ULTRA can only authorise the transplant if the relationship can be proven. The doctors looking after both the potential recipient and donor have to prepare a report for ULTRA to support the proposed reason for the transplant. An independent third party specialist doctor, who is not involved with the care of either the recipient or the donor, will also need to submit a report. This doctor must interview both parties separately and together to prepare the report. A translator may be used if necessary. The reports need to be supported by documentary evidence such as a marriage certificate, photographs of the donor and recipient together, or evidence of co-habitation.

It is illegal to buy or sell kidneys for transplant. There must be no pressure on any potential donor to donate, or recipient to accept. It is also illegal to offer money to enable the live transplant to take place.

Who can have a live kidney transplant?

Any person being considered for a cadaveric kidney transplant can be considered for live donor transplant. The criteria for acceptance for live and cadaveric transplants are the same.

The cause of the patient's kidney failure is taken into account when considering the option of live donor transplant. Recipients and donors must be fully informed of any likelihood that the recipient's original kidney disease may recur following a live donor transplant. They should also be given a realistic estimate of the long term outcome.

A person who has already had a cadaveric transplant will be able to have a live related transplant or a live unrelated transplant. But most kidney doctors would recommend that, if a live transplant is possible, it should be your first transplant. These are better, healthier kidneys – and the first transplant usually lasts the longest. So it is logical to have the best kidney first.

Can I have a live kidney transplant before I need to start dialysis?

If your kidney failure is diagnosed at an early stage, you could be considered for live kidney transplant up to six months before you need dialysis. At this point your creatinine level is likely to be about 400 micromoles/litre. If you already have a transplant that is starting to fail, you could have a live transplant before you need to return to dialysis. But this is up to your own renal unit's individual policy.

Could I donate one of my kidneys to a friend without them knowing?

It is not possible to donate a kidney anonymously. No live donor transplant will be performed without the co-operation and knowledge of both recipient and donor. The donor must be willing to donate and the recipient must also be willing to accept the kidney.

I have been told I will need dialysis in about six months time. But I would prefer a living transplant before dialysis. How can I find out if any of my family or friends are suitable donors? I've had lots of offers.

Sometimes, when a person is told they will need a transplant to treat kidney failure, they can be inundated with offers from family and friends who want to donate their kidneys.

Before a live transplant can take place, the donor needs to be carefully assessed to ensure he or she is medically suitable. This is to make sure the donor is fit enough to endure the operation and remain fit after it.

During the first assessment, the doctor will review the donor's full past medical history. If there are no medical problems, the donor will then have some simple blood tests to find out what blood group they are and test the function of the kidneys. If these are OK, the donor must then have a more detailed assessment and further investigations.

Donors' tests and investigations are held in stages. They are able to move onto the next stage of tests only after they have passed the tests of the stage before. There are five or more stages, and a complete assessment can take 3–6 months. So if you are considering a living transplant, your unit needs to start working on it now.

All potential donors must be informed that the assessment could uncover problems they did not know existed. If any medical problems are discovered with the donor, they will be told immediately. The tests can either be stopped, temporarily suspended while the medical problem is treated and resolved, or continued with any risks being discussed with donor and recipient.

What sort of people can donate one of their kidneys?

Almost anyone can donate a kidney to a loved one. However, there are some situations where live kidney donation would not be possible. These include people with the following conditions:

    (i) HIV or AIDS-related infection;
   (ii) major heart or breathing problems;
  (iii) diabetes (either type);
  (iv) significant kidney disease;
   (v) most cancers;
  (vi) very high blood pressure;
 (vii) intravenous drug abuse;
(viii) pregnancy;
  (ix) having only one kidney;
   (x) evidence of financial or non-financial coercion;
  (xi) inability of a potential donor to give informed consent.

In addition, doctors would think very seriously before allowing anyone to donate a kidney if any of the following apply:

   (i) age over 70 years;
  (ii) age below 18 years;
 (iii) intellectual impairment but able to give informed consent;
 (iv) obesity;
  (v) smoking;
 (vi) family history of diabetes;
(vii) psychiatric disorders;
(viii) hepatitis B or C infection.

There may also be situations where the cause of the recipient's kidney failure is an illness which has a higher than normal likelihood of occurring in a blood relative. Systemic lupus erythematosus is one example. In such cases, a blood relative would not be advised to donate a kidney.

Both my sister (aged 23) and my dad (aged 54) are willing to give me a kidney. Both have had all the tests and both are suitable. Which should I take? I am 28 years old and on PD.

What a difficult choice! Results are generally better from donors who are closer in age to you but, as you are young and live transplants don't always last forever, you may need two or more transplants in your life. So, on balance, it would probably be better to accept the kidney from your father while he is still relatively young, and save your sister's generous offer for later in your life (and hers) if you ever need another one.

What medical tests will I need before I can donate my kidney? My brother needs a transplant.

If your blood group is suitable, you will need to have blood tests to measure your kidney function, liver function and other things such as your haemoglobin level. These all need to be normal.

You must have an ECG (a heart trace, see page 133) and a chest X-ray to ensure there are no problems with your heart or breathing. You may also be given an 'exercise tolerance test' to see how your heart reacts under light exercise. Your blood pressure must be normal. If it is found to be higher than normal the doctors will monitor it for 24 hours as it may only be high at certain times of day or under certain circumstances.

It is important to ensure (using an ultrasound scan) that you have two kidneys. A renogram test, in which photographs of the kidney are taken a few hours after drinking a harmless radio-active dye, can confirm that both kidneys are doing equal amounts of work.

Your blood will be tested for infections such as HIV, hepatitis B and C. Your genetic make-up ('tissue type') will also be assessed. This is undertaken in live transplantation to find out if the donor and recipient are well matched. It is also necessary for live related transplants so the genetic relationship between donor and recipient can be proven.

In addition there will be a cross-match test, between donor and recipient. As with cadaveric transplantation, a negative cross-match means the transplant preparation can continue, but if the cross-match is positive, the transplant cannot go ahead.

Finally, to help the surgeons decide which kidney to remove (left or right), the blood vessels to each kidney are examined using either a CT scan or an angiogram. (Details of these procedures and the risks involved are given on pages 86–88.) This may be done a day or two before the transplant operation.

Recipient and donor will both need to have a full clinical examination. This is usually done by both the doctor looking after the patients and the surgeon who will perform the operation. It is also necessary to perform a psychological assessment of both donor and recipient. This is to make sure both are happy and understand about the procedure and the effects it may have on them and their families. The psychologist or counsellor will make sure both individuals are able to cope if the transplant fails or if anything happens to either of them.

Once a live donor has been found, how long will it be before the operation can go ahead?

The length of time it takes to prepare the donor and recipient for a live kidney transplant can vary from one unit to another, depending upon a variety of factors.

   (i) The process will be quicker if there is a full time dedicated live transplant co-ordinator.

  (ii) The process may be delayed if it is necessary for either donor or recipient to have additional pre transplant tests as a result of initial screening.

 (iii) If the donor is not a blood relative of the recipient, it will be necessary to contact ULTRA for permission to carry out the operation. This usually takes about five working days once the relevant paperwork is in order (which may take considerably longer).

On average it can take around 3–6 months to prepare for live transplant. Sometimes the time is deliberately long so as to give both parties sufficient time for careful consideration. On occasions, it can be 'rushed through' in a couple of weeks if there is urgent need for a transplant.

How is the kidney removed from the donor in a live transplant?

There are two ways a live kidney can be donated, either laparoscopically (using keyhole surgery) or open surgery. The removal of a kidney is called a nephrectomy.

- **Open nephrectomy**
  Open surgery is the usual method of removing the kidney. The surgeon makes a cut from the middle point of the side of the chest right to the side of the abdomen. Part of a rib may also need to be removed. This method leaves a large scar that can be difficult to cover up. It also takes longer for the donor to recover after the operation. However using conventional surgery significantly reduces the risk of complications during the operation.

- **Laparoscopic nephrectomy**
  Some renal units remove the kidney using keyhole surgery. A small cut is made below the tummy button. The kidney is located and removed with the assistance of a small camera that helps the surgeon to see inside the body without cutting the patient right open. The benefit of this procedure is that the patient has a smaller scar and a quicker recovery time. But there are disadvantages. There is an increased risk of complications such as potential damage to the kidney being donated.

Whichever method is used to remove the kidney, the surgeon takes great care not to damage the organ in any way. It is also important for the surgeon to remove the blood vessels and tubes surrounding the kidney, so they can be used for the recipient.

How long will I be in hospital for after donating my kidney for a live transplant? When can I return to work?

If your kidney is removed using laparoscopic nephrectomy, you will be in hospital for about 3–5 days, but after open surgery this could be 6–9 days.

How soon you return to work will depend on the type of work and your general fitness before the operation. If your work is physically demanding, you will probably need a longer recovery time than someone who has sedentary work.

If you donate your kidney by laparoscopic nephrectomy, you can probably return to work within 3–4 weeks of the operation. With open surgery it is advisable to remain off work for about 12 weeks.

I would like to donate one of my kidneys to my brother, but I'm worried about the risks of the operation.

While any surgical procedure carries with it a small risk (there is about a 1 in 2,000 risk of dying as a result of an operation), the risks to a healthy donor should be minimal if all the pre-operative tests have been carried out. You should be aware however that the more invasive tests do themselves carry some risk (see pages 84–89). Anyone who donates a kidney will be seen regularly after the operation. Most units recommend kidney donors should be seen by a kidney specialist every year for life. There is some evidence to suggest that kidney donors live longer than other people on average. Nobody knows why this might be so – maybe they look after themselves better knowing they have lost an organ.

There will be some pain and discomfort after the operation, which should get better after a few days. One in 25 patients, however, get long-term pain in the site of the wound. This can usually be controlled by intermittent injections.

Some donors may suffer from protein in their urine (proteinuria) after the operation and about 10% of all donors may develop high blood pressure. This is the same as the incidence of high blood pressure within the general population.

A major problem of donating a kidney to a loved one is the potential emotional upset if a live transplant fails at an early stage.

A friend wishes to donate me a kidney but her employer won't pay sick pay while she is off work. Is there anything I can do to help?

Some employers interpret kidney donation as self-inflicted injury and won't pay sick leave. If this is the employer's policy, there is little the employee can do. However if this is the case for your friend, it is legally acceptable (under the Human Organ Transplants Act) for her loss of earnings to be reimbursed – either by you as the recipient or by your family. Some health authorities may also reimburse these costs, but this is not the case everywhere. Ask your social worker.

If your donor is travelling from overseas solely to donate a kidney, her return airfare, together with any potential loss of earnings, should be reimbursed.

Can I choose the hospital where I have my live kidney transplant?

Although it should be possible to have the operation anywhere, it is usually performed in the recipient's own renal unit or linked transplant centre. Transplants are almost always done in a registered NHS transplant unit due to the specialist nature of the operation and its aftercare.

If you are not entitled to NHS treatment it may be possible to have a live kidney transplant privately in the UK. There are only a few centres within the UK that perform transplants privately and all foreseeable costs must be met prior to the transplant procedure.

I am 67 years old and I would like to donate a kidney to my son who has just been diagnosed with kidney failure. Am I too old?

There is no limit on the age of a live kidney donor, as long as you fulfil all the medical fitness criteria associated with live donor suitability (see page 156).

I was diagnosed with kidney failure six months ago and started dialysis straightaway. At first, I thought I could wait for a cadaveric transplant, but now I have been on dialysis for so long I don't think I can. How do I go about asking my family if they would like to donate a kidney to me?

Unfortunately you are the only person who can ask a friend or relative to donate a kidney to you. The renal unit cannot ask on your behalf. However, when you have your initial transplant assessment with the transplant doctor, live transplantation should be discussed. It may be possible to invite your relative or friend along to this appointment with you, but explain that you are interested in having a live kidney transplant beforehand.

Once your relatives and friends know they could become donors, they may automatically volunteer.

I've been told I'm a good match for donating a kidney to my sister. What will happen if I change my mind about the operation and don't donate?

If you decide not to donate your kidney, your sister will have to wait for a cadaveric transplant. This could take many years and it may never happen. It is also possible her health may deteriorate if she stays on dialysis for a long time. However, your offer of a kidney is entirely your decision and you should not feel pressured into giving it.

I am a diabetic in kidney failure. Can my donor donate his kidney and pancreas?

No. Your donor has two kidneys and can live quite healthily with just one. But we all have just one pancreas and your donor cannot live without it.

My brother would like to donate his kidney to me but he lives in India. Could the transplant be done in the UK or should I go to India?

The best option would be for you to have the operation in the UK. Your brother will need to come to the UK for all the tests to make sure he is a suitable donor. He will also need to stay for about three months after the operation to ensure he has made a full recovery. All the criteria for live transplantation remain the same as described on page 156.

If you are eligible for NHS care, there will be no charge made for your operation and aftercare, or for your brother's.

You could travel to India for the operation, but this will be costly and there may be an increased risk of infection or other complications after the operation.

My partner and I are gay. He would like to donate one of his kidneys to me. Can he do this?

Yes, provided your blood groups and cross match are compatible. You will both need to have all the same tests that are carried out for heterosexual unrelated donors, including gaining permission from ULTRA and health and fitness tests.

My friend has been told she has three kidneys. Can she safely donate one to me?

She could if she has three healthy kidneys. However, most people with three kidneys have three small kidneys, none of which would be suitable for donation.

Will there be a risk of rejection after a live transplant?

Unless your live transplant has come from a genetically identical donor (an identical twin), there will be a risk of rejecting the kidney. It is important you take your immunosuppressant medication to help avoid this problem.

My husband will be donating his kidney to me soon. Is it true that if we have more sex before the operation, there will be less risk of rejecting the kidney?

This is a myth. There is no evidence that partners who have had an active sex life before the transplant have any less risk of rejection than those who don't.

I had a live transplant from my mother about eight years ago, which failed last year. I know my sister is a suitable donor as she was tested at the same time as my mother. Could I have her kidney now?

Yes, you could have your sister's kidney so long as the usual criteria are fulfilled.

Drugs and transplants

I've recently had a kidney transplant. My doctor has put me on an anti-TB drug. Why?

When you have a transplant you need to take two or three drugs that prevent your body from rejecting the new kidney. These are called immunosuppressant drugs, and they also make your body less able to fight off infections.

If you or a member of your close family have had TB (tuberculosis – a long term infection, usually of the lungs), you will need to take an anti-TB drug to prevent you from developing TB now. If you are Asian, you may also be given this treatment.

You will only need to take it for up to a year while you are taking higher doses of your immunosuppressant drugs.

Isoniazid is the drug usually prescribed. It has some rare but unpleasant side effects. It can cause liver problems, which will show up on your blood tests. It can also cause peripheral neuropathy (loss of feeling in your arms and legs). Taking a vitamin called Pyridoxine once a day can prevent this problem.

What is the best regimen of immunosuppressant drugs for my new kidney?

All patients who have a kidney transplant need to take immunosuppressant drugs. The aim is to dampen down your immune system sufficiently to stop your body rejecting the transplant kidney, while still keeping it active enough to fight any infections in your body. Finding the balance can be difficult.

There is no 'best' regimen. Different patients need different combinations of drugs, and different dosages. A good regimen is one that suits you, preventing kidney rejection while having relatively few side effects.

The most commonly used immunosuppressants are currently cyclosporin, azathioprine and prednisolone (a steroid). Newer drugs, such as tacrolimus (FK506) and mycophenolate, are also becoming available.

The aim of newer immunosuppressants is to make transplants last longer. But their use is controversial. They are generally stronger than existing drugs, suppressing the immune system to a greater degree. This may explain why serious side effects, such as diabetes or lymphoma, are more common with these drugs. It is thought this is how they make kidneys last longer, by reducing the likelihood and severity of rejection. However, if they do make transplants last longer, it is not yet clear that the 'extra kidney-life' gained is very long or whether the side effects are worth it.

Do I have to take the immunosuppressant drugs every day, forever?

It is vital for you to take the two or three different kinds of

immunosuppressant drugs every day, forever or until the kidney
fails. If you stop taking the drugs, your immune system starts
'fighting back'. If you are unable to take your immunosuppressants, either because they have run out or because you
are suffering from diarrhoea or vomiting, you should go to the
hospital at once. Your immune system does not forget there is a
'foreign' kidney in the body. It is always waiting for a chance to
attack and reject it.

**What are the common side effects of the immuno-
suppressant drugs I have to take?**

There are lots of side effects from immunosuppressant drugs. All
of the most commonly used immunosuppressants have major
problems.

- **Cyclosporin**
  This is the most important drug used to prevent kidney
  rejection. Unfortunately, if you are given too much of it,
  cyclosporin is toxic to the kidney and can prevent the
  transplant from working (a condition known as 'cyclosporin
  toxicity'). You might ask why doctors readily prescribe a
  drug to help the kidney, which can itself damage the kidney.
      At present though, there is no drug that is clearly better
  than cyclosporin. To reduce the risk of cyclosporin toxicity,
  the amount of the drug in your blood is monitored regularly.
  If problems do occur, these can usually be reversed by
  reducing the dose or stopping the drug completely.
      Cyclosporin can also damage your liver.
      Another side effect is a condition called gum hypertrophy
  – an excessive growth of your gums, which can be unsightly.
  It is less likely to develop if you practise good dental
  hygiene, including regular flossing between the teeth.
  Cyclosporin sometimes causes excessive growth of hair on
  the face and body, which can be distressing. It can also
  cause diabetes, which can require insulin.
      If the side effects of cyclosporin are severe, tacrolimus
  may be used in its place. Some renal units use tacrolimus

from the start of the transplant. This is controversial as it has a greater tendency to cause lymphoma, which can be extremely serious, and diabetes.

When taking cyclosporin you should avoid grapefruit juice for one hour before taking a dose because it affects the way it gets into the body. Many other medicines affect the way this drug works – always check with your doctor or pharmacist before taking anything.

Cyclosporin comes as different types or brands. You should always take the same brand and not swap. It is sometimes called 'Cy . A'.

• Azathioprine

Unfortunately, azathioprine can suppress blood cell production in your bone marrow, where blood cells are made. This can lead to a number of serious problems. If too few red blood cells are produced, you will suffer from **anaemia** causing tiredness. If there are too few white blood cells, you will develop a condition called **neutropenia** in which your ability to fight infection is reduced. If too few platelets are produced, you may develop **thrombo-cytopenia**, which makes you bleed more easily.

If you are taking azathioprine, you may suffer from any or all of the above problems. Stopping the drug or reducing the dose will normally put matters right. Azathioprine can also damage your liver.

Some renal units use another drug, mycophenylate, instead of azathioprine. However, this can have similar side effects, especially neutropenia. It may be a question of seeing which drug is best suited to a particular patient.

• Prednisolone

This drug is a steroid and like other steroid drugs, it can cause thinning of your skin leading to easy bruising, and facial swelling giving a red and rounded appearance to your face. These problems may lessen if the dose is reduced.

Taking prednisolone can also cause diabetes. At worst, this might mean you will have to take tablets or give yourself insulin injections – perhaps for the rest of your life or until the kidney fails.

While taking prednisolone, you are more likely to develop infections, especially during periods of stress. You should report any infection to your doctor. If you or anyone in your circle catches chicken pox, tell your doctor immediately but don't stop taking your prednisolone. You should also contact your doctor if you develop chicken pox within three months of stopping prednisolone.

In some patients, prednisolone can cause bone weakness, which may eventually lead to crumbling of the joints, especially the hip joints. This can occur within a year of a transplant. Replacement of one or both of your hips may become necessary.

After my first transplant I had cyclosporin. This time I have been given tacrolimus. The doctor tells me there are fewer side effects. Is this true?

Tacrolimus and cyclosporin are both immunosuppressant drugs, and both have side effects although they are not the same for each drug. So side effects are not fewer, though they may be different.

Unlike cyclosporin, tacrolimus is unlikely to cause swelling of the gums or excess hair growth, but it can cause pins and needles in your arms and increase your chance of developing diabetes and lymphoma.

All immunosuppressants make you more likely to develop infections and to become more ill with them than other people. You should report any infections to your doctor.

The levels of drugs will be monitored in clinic because, like cyclosporin, too much tacrolimus can damage your kidney. When you come to clinic, do not take your morning dose until after you have had your blood taken.

Grapefruit juice and food should be avoided for an hour before your dose. Other drugs may cause problems with tacrolimus – always check with your doctor or pharmacist before taking any other medicines. Tacrolimus used to be known as FK506, so you may hear it called 'FK'.

My son has just received a transplant, and been put on lots of tablets. The doctor says that, because he is taking azathioprine, they have to keep a close eye on his blood results. Why is this?

Azathioprine is an immunosuppressant drug which works by reducing the number of white cells (the ones that fight off infection) in the blood. If the doctors give your son too much azathioprine, he will not have enough white cells left to fight off even very minor infections. So the number of white cells in his blood must be monitored regularly. If the level of white cells reduces too far, the dose will have to be reduced, or even stopped.

Your son will probably be advised to take his azathioprine as a single dose after his evening meal. Common side effects (which can be reduced by taking the tablets with food) include feeling sick, vomiting and loss of appetite. Other rare, more serious side effects include fever and rashes. Problems with the blood, liver or kidney may also occur.

Azathioprine is sometimes called 'Aza' for short.

My daughter has a kidney transplant, and is on prednisolone. She is tired all the time and seems to have put on a lot of weight. Should she change drugs?

As well as being an immunosuppressant drug, prednisolone is a steroid. Weight gain, fattening of the face, and tiredness are all common side effects. Over a longer period of time, prednisolone can also cause acne and damage the hip joints. If diabetes occurs, your daughter may need to have insulin injections.

Most people start with a high dose of prednisolone after a transplant. If all goes well, this will be reduced fairly quickly over the next few months. The risks of side effects are higher if you take more of the drug, so as time goes by and the dose is reduced these risks also reduce. But talk to your doctor sooner rather than later if you are worried.

Some people will need to take a small dose of prednisolone for as long as the transplant works. This small dose is usually not enough to cause weight gain or a moon face but can cause other side effects (described above).

I have just had a second transplant and have been put on a drug called mycophenolate. I have never heard of this. What is it?

Mycophenolate is similar in action to azathioprine, which you may have had with your first transplant.

Your recommended daily dose should be taken in two equal doses, morning and night.

The most common side effects of mycophenolate include diarrhoea, feeling sick, headaches and dizziness. Other side effects include a fall in the number of white cells in the blood (as with azathioprine). This will be checked for by regular blood tests.

As with any immunosuppressant drug you are more likely to develop infections and any infections you get may be worse than normal. You should report any signs of infection to your doctor. Some other drugs may cause problems with mycophenolate – always check with your doctor or pharmacist before taking any new medicine.

I have had a transplant and have been given a lozenge to suck once a day. Why? I don't have a sore throat.

In the first few months after a transplant while you are on high doses of immunosuppressant drugs, you are more likely to develop infections. One of the common infections is thrush or candida, a fungal infection which affects the mouth. If sucked once a day, amphotericin lozenges can help to prevent you getting this infection.

The lozenges are best sucked about 15 minutes after a meal. Food and drink should be avoided for one hour afterwards.

I have just had a transplant and, among other drugs, I have been given Co-trimoxazole. What is this?

In the first few months after a transplant, while you are on high doses of immunosuppressant drugs, you are more likely to develop infections. One common problem is a specific chest infection, which Co-trimoxazole can help to prevent. It also helps to stop urine infections. The tablets are taken once a day.

Common side effects of Co-trimoxazole include nausea and skin rashes. If the tablets make you feel sick, try taking them with food. If you develop a rash you should report it to your doctor straightaway. More rare side effects include problems with your blood or liver, which should show up on blood tests.

7

Living with kidney failure

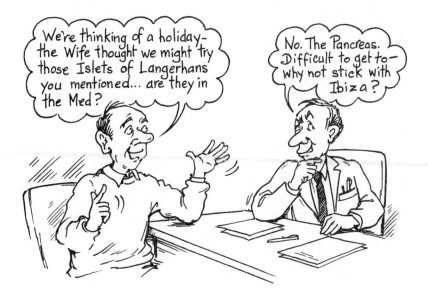

Being diagnosed with kidney failure need not necessarily be the end of a positive and enjoyable life. This chapter looks at some of the ways your quality of life can be maintained at home, at work and in your leisure time.

Holidays and travel

I will have to start dialysis in the next six months. My wife and I used to go for holidays all the time. Should we continue? Can you give me some general advice?

Going on holiday when you are on dialysis is not only possible but highly recommended. Most patients will be actively encouraged to do this by the renal unit team who will help with the arrangements.

It is essential to check with your unit before planning or booking anything.

Travel for kidney patients on dialysis does require more planning, so last minute bookings are not a realistic option. However, the limitations as to type of holiday and holiday locations are far fewer than you might imagine. The Internet is a wonderful source of information and advice – see, for example, kidneywise.com, and kidneypatientguide.org. The globaldialysis. com website includes a full list of renal units worldwide, details of kidney patient associations and charities around the world, plus lots of other useful information and links for the travelling kidney patient. There is also an organisation called Eurodial, based in France, which publishes a comprehensive directory of units around the world in booklet format and on the web.

If you have a transplant, you will still need to do a lot of planning. You will need a letter from the hospital confirming you are fit to travel, to secure travel insurance; advice on immunisation; and a supply of all your tablets. It is a good idea to take a written list of your tablets, including the doses and how often you have to take them.

Choosing your destination
Whatever your treatment, it makes sense to ensure you are within reasonable reach of medical support in case of emergencies. A beach holiday in Spain may be safer than trekking in Nepal.

Choosing accommodation

Check that the accommodation you are considering can cope with any special requirements you may have. For example, if it is a hotel, do they cater for special diets? Certain UK charities – such as the National Kidney Federation and British Kidney Patient Association – can help find suitable holiday accommodation for kidney patients.

Holiday insurance

If you are going to a country outside the European Union (such as the USA) it is better not to book your holiday until you have taken out holiday insurance that covers you for a pre-existing medical condition. Most standard policies do not.

I am on PD. Should I still take holidays?

Holidays are a great way to reinforce the fact that you can still enjoy the good things in life as a kidney patient – and they also provide a welcome break for carers. However, there are a number of things to organise before you go. The following tips may be useful

(i) **Think ahead**
It takes some planning to make sure your treatment requirements go smoothly while you are away. Leave yourself plenty of time between starting the planning process and the time you would like to be away. Inevitably, more exotic locations often involve more planning and notice. As a general guide, you should allow a minimum of three months to make the necessary arrangements. A shorter amount of notice may be possible, depending on your destination.

(ii) **Delivery of supplies**
Dialysis fluid can be delivered to a wide range of destinations around the world. This will be arranged through the company who manufactures it, and your renal unit will help ensure this is co-ordinated for you.

The notice required for delivery can be up to eight weeks, so advance planning is important.

Make sure you call the destination two or three days before departure to check supplies have arrived safely. Take the name of the person you speak to and ask where the supplies are being stored, and where they will be when you arrive, especially if you are likely to arrive late at night or early in the morning when a skeleton staff may be on duty.

Make sure you know who to contact if you find there are any bags or ancillary items missing when you arrive. This is extremely rare and if it should occur, the company concerned will do whatever is necessary to get you what you need urgently.

(iii) **Assistance at ports, airports, etc.**
If you tire easily or have problems with mobility, most airports now offer wheelchairs and/or chauffeured 'buggies', which will whisk you through check-in, departure procedures and passport control in minutes. Ferry ports, railway stations and many special attractions also offer this type of assistance. You will need to book this in advance – your travel agent should be able to help you or you can simply ring direct to see what help is available and book your buggy.

(iv) **Insurance of APD machines**
None of the holiday insurance companies will provide cover for APD machines. It should usually be possible to arrange cover through the insurance company you use to cover household contents.

(v) **Customs**
Ask your doctor for a letter confirming that your APD machine and bags of fluid are for medical treatment. The letter should also state that the bags of fluid are not to be opened.

(vi) **Electricity supply**
For any equipment, such as APD machines, you should check the electricity voltage is compatible, and you have the correct adapters for the plugs.

(vii) **Exchanges during the journey**
You should always discuss your travel itinerary with your PD nurse, who will advise you on the most suitable exchange plan for your outward and return journeys. If you need to carry out an exchange at the airport or port terminal, ask to use either the medical room or the St John's Ambulance treatment room for your exchange. If your itinerary means you won't have to carry out an exchange until you reach your destination, it is still advisable to carry one dialysis bag in your hand luggage in case of delays.

(viii) **Cleanliness**
You should avoid carrying out exchanges in unhygienic or cramped areas, such as plane toilets. Don't take risks, you can catch up with your exchanges later in a safe, clean environment. If you are on CAPD, it will do you no harm to do three exchanges on the day of travel, if you usually do four. Most people actually take more care with their exchanges when in a different environment, and the percentage of people who get peritonitis when on holiday is very small.

I am a haemodialysis patient. Are there any special things for me to think about if I want to travel abroad?

It is a little more difficult for haemodialysis patients to arrange a holiday, but this should not deter you. The first thing you need to do is find a haemodialysis unit. This may mean you need to be a little more flexible in terms of choice of destination, since you will need to be in easy reach of a unit which can accommodate you. There are plenty of exotic locations with haemodialysis units, and even special cruises designed for dialysis patients.

The Internet is useful for finding a unit. As well as its directory and booklets, Eurodial (see above) also has a travel agency that can help with recommending accommodation, arranging insurance, and booking your holiday. Globaldialysis has a list of renal units all over the world, as well as other useful information. If you plan to visit a European country, make sure the unit you choose is not a private facility, for which you will have to pay. Ask if they accept the E111 (see facing page). Many European units that advertise holiday dialysis, are in fact wholly private, profit making concerns. Make sure you are aware of any costs involved for your dialysis while you are on holiday. Some countries have reciprocal arrangements with the UK for dialysis (including the countries covered by E111). However, since the reciprocal agreements allow UK citizens the same care as would be provided to the citizens of the country you are visiting, there may be certain costs for which you will be liable. These may include transport and the cost of any drugs prescribed during your visit. Some health authorities may contribute to the cost of dialysis abroad.

If you are visiting Spain, you will need a special Spanish form called a P10, which you should obtain before leaving the UK. Your renal unit will organise this for you.

Keep your renal unit advised of any research you are doing for your holiday – they may need to give you certain criteria (eg infection control policy) for your needs in your 'holiday' unit. Bear in mind there may be slight differences in the equipment and procedures used by the unit you visit. You could discuss what these might be with your 'home' renal unit in advance, so you are not taken unawares. Ask for a print-out of your dialysis prescription, and any problems you encounter from time to time, such as low blood pressure, problems with fistula flow etc – so you can take this with you, to give to your holiday unit. You will also need to take the results of recent tests for hepatitis B,C and HIV. It is a good idea to check that the unit you are going to isolates infectious patients.

If you tire easily, and need assistance at ports or airports, the same advice will apply as for patients on PD (see above).

Check with your renal unit for advice about swimming or any other sports you want to try while on holiday.

If I were called up for a transplant, would my holiday insurance cover me?

Your holiday insurance is unlikely to cover the cost of an early return home, unless you have specifically mentioned it in your insurance agreement. The National Kidney Federation has useful information on holiday insurance, as does the kidneywise.com website. Remember also, to let your transplant unit have a contact number when you are away. If you go abroad, you should be able to return to the UK in less than 12 hours. People have lost the opportunity of a kidney by being difficult to contact.

I often have to travel abroad on business, but rarely stay away more than one night. I am going onto haemodialysis soon. Should I change my job?

Travel is a common requirement of many jobs nowadays. There is often no reason why kidney patients should not be able to make short business trips – either in the UK or overseas. There is always a danger of being stranded abroad when you are due back for dialysis, so ensure you carry a list of haemodialysis units in Europe (available from Eurodial – see Appendix 3). Talk to your employers about whether your travel insurance covers the costs of urgent treatment abroad, and carry your Form E111 when visiting countries in the European Union.

What is Form E111?

Form E111, usually available from post offices, entitles you to the same free or subsidised hospital treatment as would be provided to citizens of the country you are visiting in the event of a minor health emergency. Be aware this means that some of the costs, for example for drugs and ambulance transport, may be payable in some countries.

E111 does not provide cover should you or any members of your family need to fly home urgently, or if you need to return from holiday because a transplant kidney becomes available.

It is a good idea to keep your E111 in a safe place, with your passport. Always keep a photocopy with the original. Countries covered by form E111 include the EU countries and some others such as Iceland. Check the form carefully to see that all countries you will visit are covered. They currently include Austria, Belgium, Denmark, Finland, France, Germany, Greece, Iceland, Italy, Ireland, Liechtenstein, Luxembourg, Netherlands, Norway, Portugal, Spain, Sweden and the UK. You can use the same E111 for as long as you remain resident in the UK, but you will need to apply for a new one if any of your children leave school.

Health Advice for Travellers is a booklet from the Department of Health, containing comprehensive information on the E111, as well as details about which healthcare costs are covered, tips on avoiding health risks and information about vaccinations required to visit certain countries.

I have been told I will need to go on dialysis in the next year. What vaccinations will I need before going to India?

The vaccination requirements for India (and every country) change each year. This is because infectious diseases come and go, so something travellers needed to be vaccinated against last year may no longer be a problem.

Ask your GP or travel agent what immunisations you will require, but check with your renal unit before having any vaccinations as some may not be recommended for kidney patients, and transplant patients have to be especially careful of vaccines (see below). You should also be aware that some anti-malarial drugs, necessary in many countries, should be taken in reduced dosage by kidney patients. Check with your doctor.

Irrespective of which airline you are using, the British Airways Travel Clinics (see Appendix 3) offer advice on keeping healthy while abroad and can help you with most of your travel health requirements. They have a team of medical staff who are happy to offer advice to anyone planning to travel, whether by land, air or sea.

The Travel Clinics receive up-to-the-minute information on 84 different health hazards in more than 250 countries, so advice can be specifically tailored to each individual journey. A comprehensive range of vaccines is available at all British Airways Travel Clinics, which are also registered Yellow Fever immunisation centres.

I've got a stable transplant, with a creatinine around 105 micromoles per litre. I am anxious about going abroad. Can you give me some general advice.

It sounds as though you have a well functioning transplant. This does not mean you cannot enjoy travel, but you do have to be sensible.

(i) **Don't forget your tablets**
   Missing out on your immunosuppressant tablets for even 24 hours can cause you to reject your kidney and lose it forever. So, take more than you need, just in case something happens to delay your return journey.

(ii) **Stay out of the sun**
   Transplant patients are three times more likely than other people to get skin cancers after a transplant because of the immunosuppressant drugs they need to take. However, there are precautions you can take to reduce your risk of skin cancer dramatically. You should keep indoors or at least in shade between 10 am and 2 pm when the sun's UV rays are strongest. When you do go out, always use a strong sunblock with an SPF (sun protection factor) of at least 25. You should also protect your skin with suitable clothing. Long-sleeved shirts (with collars) and hats are a good idea. Be aware that many summer-weight fabrics don't give enough protection and fibres like cotton offer even less protection when wet.
   It is a good idea to wear sunglasses that block 99–100 percent of UV radiation. Check the label when you buy them.
   You should also avoid using sun lamps to develop a tan before you go.
   Examine your skin regularly. If you find any unusual blemishes or moles, especially one that changes in size, shape or colour, see your doctor.

(iii) **Avoid infections**

Transplant immunosuppressant drugs reduce your ability to fight infections. Simple precautions include:

- avoid contact with people who have a cold, flu or any infectious disease such as chickenpox;
- don't drink local water in poorly developed countries – boil the water or buy bottled water;
- avoid salads unless you have washed them yourself, and avoid ice cubes unless you have made them from bottled water;
- avoid ice cream from street vendors;
- avoid travelling to countries where the risk of catching an infection is high – MASTA and British Airways Clinics (see Appendix 3) can advise you.

(iv) **Immunisations**

Make sure you have been appropriately vaccinated before you travel. The immunosuppressant drugs you need to take after a transplant make it unsafe for you to receive certain vaccines. These are the 'live' vaccines, which include: TB, rubella, measles, mumps, oral typhoid and oral polio. Check with your renal unit about which vaccinations you can and can't have.

Malaria prevention tablets are needed for travel to certain areas of the world. They are required before you travel, while you are away and for four weeks after you return. Most of these can be taken safely with immunosuppressant drugs, but the appropriate dose for you will depend on your kidney function.

Immunisation advice can be obtained at your local GP clinic or at any of the British Airways Travel Clinics.

What should I do with my medications?

It is safest to divide your supply of tablets. Keep half with you in your hand luggage, and pack the other half in the luggage you check in, or give it to a companion to carry.

You will need a letter from your doctor stating that the drugs you are carrying are prescription drugs.

It is helpful to carry a written list of all the details of your medications, including: the prescription names (as written on the label), the dosages and how often you take them – so that if your supply is lost, you can advise doctors accordingly.

If you need to take medication that must be kept cool, pack it in a small picnic cool bag or a jiffy bag with ice packs, or use a wide neck thermos flask which has been chilled. EPO does not need refrigeration for journeys of up to six hours, but make sure you allow time for transfers and delays when calculating the length of your journey.

On your return trip, remember to declare to customs any drugs you were given or prescribed.

I'm off camping in the South of France. Should I take a first aid kit?

It is worth taking a basic first aid kit, including an emergency supply of plasters, bandages, antiseptic cream, painkillers, syringes/needles, insect repellent, insect bite ointment and anti-diarrhoea tablets.

My wife and I always feel that one of the great pleasures of travelling is sampling the local food. But now I am on dialysis. Is it safe for me to eat whatever I want while abroad?

Remember you are on holiday, and need to have fun! The food and drink in developed countries is just as safe, or safer, than ours, but you should be careful about what you eat and drink in less developed countries. Before you go, talk to your dietitian about local foods to avoid. If you are travelling by plane, ask your travel agent to advise the airline of special dietary requirements.

A sensible precaution in less developed countries is to use only bottled water – for drinking, making ice cubes and brushing your teeth. It is not advisable to buy ice cream from street vendors. Try to avoid salads and fruit that does not need peeling, unless you can wash them in bottled water. Fruit you need to peel ('wrapped by nature') is generally safer.

Do I have to pay particular attention to sun protection? I'm off to Spain tomorrow.

Dialysis patients need to take all the normal precautions: make sure you take a high factor sunscreen with you, and avoid over-exposure to sunlight. Sun protection is particularly important for transplant patients (see page 179). Wear long-sleeved shirts and a hat, and remember that the sun can burn you through water or clouds.

This will be my first holiday since I became ill and I'm a bit nervous. What do I do in event of an emergency?

Make sure you and your travelling companion(s) have emergency contact numbers with you at all times. These should include the telephone numbers of the nearest renal unit to your destination, your UK renal unit, travel agent and insurance company.

Is there any help with the cost of holidays?

Some patients and carers may get charitable help from one of the Kidney Associations towards the cost of their holiday. The BKPA has its own holiday centres, and may help with funding either to one of these or other destinations. Your renal social worker can help you apply. Some local KPAs also have holiday dialysis facilities, which may be available at a subsidised rate, or they may offer financial help towards the cost of your holiday.

My wife (who is on PD) and I want to spend a long week-end in the Peak District. How can we do this?

If you are taking a car, you can probably pack enough bags in the boot to take with you. You could then do your exchanges at your hotel, or in the car if you were out for the day. PD patients have successfully dialysed on camping holidays, on narrow boats and sailing holidays – in fact almost anywhere. So, don't feel you are restricted in the sort of holiday you can choose. If you would prefer not to carry the bags with you, ask your PD nurse to arrange a delivery of fluid to the place where you will be staying. This can be arranged provided you give several weeks notice.

My father-in-law wants to visit the UK. He is from India but is a British Citizen. He requires haemodialysis three times a week. Will there be a charge for this and does he need to book in advance?

If he is a British Citizen, there should not be a charge. It is essential he books in advance. Dialysis units cannot fit holiday patients into their schedules without proper notice.

My son (who is on haemodialysis) and I are going to Turkey on holiday. Do I need to mention my son's illness to the travel insurance company?

You certainly do. If there were any emergency due to his condition, you would not be covered. Recently a patient, who had not declared his renal failure on his travel insurance, was taken ill on a plane which was diverted to the nearest airport close to a hospital. He received a bill for the cost of diverting the plane – £30,000!

Where can I get holiday insurance and how do I check if I'm covered as a CAPD patient?

This is a common question. Holiday insurance is hard, but not impossible, to find. And it can be expensive. The National Kidney Federation will put you in touch with an insurance company sympathetic to the needs of renal patients. When applying for cover, make sure you state on the form the type of dialysis you receive.

Are there any risks to having haemodialysis abroad?

In some parts of the world, including parts of the Indian Subcontinent and the Middle East, there is a high incidence of hepatitis B and C in haemodialysis units. Hepatitis can make you very unwell, or even kill you. It can also affect your chances of getting a transplant. PD may be a safer option in these countries.

We've been planning to visit my brother in Australia, but now my husband has been diagnosed with kidney failure and told he will need dialysis in three months. Should we still go?

There is no reason why you should not go if he is well. It will be easier for you both to go before he needs dialysis, rather than afterwards. But do check with his doctor that he is safe to travel. Remember too that your holiday insurance will have to cover emergency dialysis, if his kidneys deteriorate while you are away.

Eating, drinking and socialising

Why are high levels of potassium in the blood bad for me? My dietitian has ruled out some of my favourite foods. I'm on haemodialysis.

A high blood potassium can cause problems with your nerves and muscles and ultimately may affect your heart. Many foods which are high in potassium can be included in the diet but you will need to discuss with your dietitian how to do this safely.

We have a very busy social life and I am often out during the week at lunches. How can I keep up with my diet while I am out?

There is no reason why you can't keep up with your diet, you just need to choose carefully. Here are some examples that might help:

  (i) avoid lots of gravy and sauces, this will help you control your fluid intake;
 (ii) keep to small portions of vegetables and try to stick to the lower potassium varieties;

(iii) rice, pasta, noodles and breads are all good choices because they are low in potassium;

(iv) don't add salt to your food and ask the waiter/chef if it is possible to use less when they prepare your meal;

(v) include the fruit and vegetables that you eat out as part of your daily allowances;

(vi) avoid salted snacks and savouries served with drinks (nuts, crisps, sausage rolls);

(vii) avoid fruit and vegetable juices. Cordials with a low fruit content are more suitable. Spirits will give you less fluid and potassium than wines and beers.

I don't feel overweight but the doctor says that I am. Why is important to keep to an ideal weight?

It is important not to be too fat or too thin. Being too fat can lead to problems with blood pressure, your joints, blood fats and heart disease. If you are too thin then you may not be taking enough of the important nutrients. This will make you more likely to develop infections and take longer to recover from them.

It is a good idea to check with your dietitian to agree what weight you should aim for. As a general rule, you should:

(i) eat three regular meals a day, including breakfast;

(ii) take regular activity – ask your doctor to recommend suitable forms of exercise for you;

(iii) eat sensibly. Avoid fatty and sugary foods and don't add extra sugar or salt to your food. Instead, include more starchy foods (potato, bread, rice or pasta) at each meal.

Since my transplant I have put on lots of weight. My friend has some slimming tablets, do they work and are they alright to use with kidney failure?

There are no quick fixes when it comes to losing weight. Medication to help lose weight may be obtained on prescription from your doctor in special cases. However like the rest of us, you will need to make permanent changes to your diet and lifestyle to control your weight permanently. Always check with your renal doctor or renal pharmacist before you take any non-prescription medications.

I'm on haemodialysis. Most of the time I try to keep to my diet and fluid restrictions, but every now and then I feel 'why shouldn't I have what I want for a change?' The nurses nag me about coming in with too much fluid, but they don't know what it's like, drinking only a litre a day. I used to go to the pub and have twice that in an hour. They always have a huge box of chocolates on the desk as well, and dip in all day. They don't understand.

You are absolutely right. Nobody except another kidney patient really knows what it's like. It always seems like nagging if someone tells you what you should be doing, when you know perfectly well anyway. You can take responsibility for your own life, rather than leaving the doctors and nurses to take control. As long as you understand what you are doing, and know the reasons for fluid and other restrictions, it is really up to you to decide whether to go along with it or not. It is your life after all.

Most patients feel like you do from time to time and break the rules. The art is to break them safely and not too often. Everybody needs a treat occasionally. Learn how to treat yourself without making yourself ill.

Before I started dialysis I was told to eat less meat and other protein. Now I've started on PD the dietitian has told me to eat more protein. Why?

Different kinds of treatments and dialysis affect your body in different ways. We know that many people on PD need extra protein in their diet. One reason is that you lose a little protein each time you drain out an exchange. To help replace this loss, you may need to increase the amount of protein that you eat each day. The reason for the dietitian's change of tune is simply that diets need to change as treatment changes in kidney failure.

I am a vegetarian on PD. I am worried that my potassium intake is too high because all of the foods I eat that are good sources of protein are also high in potassium.

Many of the vegetarian sources of protein are high in potassium but fortunately PD is generally good at removing this. It should be safe to include pulses, beans, tofu, cottage cheese and quorn in the diet. These will help to provide sufficient protein.

I have been on haemodialysis for eight months. Recently people are telling me that I'm drinking too much! I've never had this problem before and I'm not drinking any more than I usually do but my weight gain between each dialysis session is getting bigger.

There are two possible reasons for this. Firstly, it is possible that you are getting a lot of fluid from the food you are eating rather than what you are drinking. Try to think whether you have been eating more liquid foods like soups, gravies or custards. If you have, you need either to cut down on these foods or account for them within your fluid allowance.

A second explanation could be that you are passing less urine now than when you started on dialysis. It is common for people's remaining kidney function to diminish once they are on dialysis. Do you feel this might be the case with you?

I feel thirsty all of the time and want to drink. I know that I shouldn't but I can't help it, what should I do?

This is a question that many people ask. It is difficult feeling that you want to drink and knowing that you can't. Here are some tips to help you:

  (i) spread your fluid allowance out through the day;
 (ii) avoid salty foods and adding salt to your food – this will only make you feel more thirsty;
(iii) use some of your fluid allowance to make ice cubes (these will be more refreshing and last longer than sips of water);

(iv) try not to have milk based drinks, as they will make your
     mouth 'sticky' and make you want to drink more (this
     may include tea and coffee);
 (v) limit the amount of sauces and gravy you have with your
     meals;
(vi) good oral hygiene will often help;
(vii) try to think why you want to drink. Is it because you are
     bored, for comfort, to be sociable?

**I am 24 years old and on haemodialysis. My social life
revolved around the 'local' and drinking pints with my
mates. Now I have to watch my fluid intake. I am too
embarrassed to tell my mates about my kidney failure, so
I don't go to the pub any more. My social life is empty
now. What can I do?**

Many renal patients feel like you do, and cut themselves off from
friends and their social network. This is unfortunate as it can lead
to increased boredom and frustration. Can you try telling them
about your kidney failure, and perhaps show them some
literature on it (maybe leaflets from your renal unit, maybe this
book)? They may then be more able to understand your
problems, especially concerning fluid intake and fluid overload.
Then you can enjoy a night out with them like before, drinking
'shorts' to keep up with them.

**I am a 30-year-old woman on haemodialysis, and go out
with the girls every Friday night. They say, 'one pint won't
hurt'. Will it? We always go for a curry afterwards. I have
to eat boiled rice, but they tempt me with Chicken Tikka
Massala, my favourite curry. They call me a wimp if I don't
eat it. What can I do?**

Experience for most of us shows that one pint leads to another,
and another. It is easy to lose sight of how much you are drinking.
Remember it will be you, and not your friends, who may become
breathless and have to go into the renal unit for an emergency
dialysis session at 2 am. Most haemodialysis patients can get fluid

overload if they drink more than their fluid restriction, which is usually less than 1 litre, or two pints, a day. Drinking shorts may be an alternative.

Eating a curry that might be high in potassium may not be a good idea, but you don't have to have boiled rice alone. Talk to your dietitian about 'low potassium' curries, like a dry vegetable curry. You may find that either you don't have a problem with potassium (ask to see your blood tests, before and after haemodialysis) and you can eat a pretty normal diet; or, if you have longer on dialysis, you can eat largely what you want.

Work and employment rights

I am due to start dialysis. Should I stop work?

Financially and psychologically, it will be better for you to remain at work if you can, even if you have to take some time off. Talk to your employers, who may be willing to let you reduce your hours for a while, or move to lighter work within the same company.

Most workplaces can accommodate a PD exchange at work. If adaptations are required for you to do this safely, there may be government funding available. If you are having haemodialysis, you may be able to negotiate with your employer a way to fit it in with your working hours, or your local unit may offer haemodialysis in the evening – or even on a night shift.

The Disability Employment Adviser at your local Job Centre can advise you further.

My employer is asking me to hand in my notice. Can I be made to leave work?

Your employer cannot make you leave your job just because you have kidney failure. Look at your contract of employment to establish what you are entitled to in terms of sick pay. If you are on long term Incapacity Benefit, your employer will have to follow employment procedures to be able to make you redundant on health grounds. If you are working for a company that employs 20 people or more, your rights are embodied in the Disability Discrimination Act (1995). Employment law is complicated. Seek help from your Union, Citizens Advice Bureau or other advisory services.

How can I get advice about employment and disability rights?

The Citizens Advice Bureau is an excellent source of advice if you feel you are being treated unfairly by your employer. They will be able to advise you, free of charge, and help you decide what your next step should be.

Solicitors specialising in employment law can also advise you, but make sure you are aware of their charges before asking a solicitor to spend time on your case. Many solicitors will give you the first half-hour's advice for a fixed sum.

Some solicitors may provide you with help and advice under the Legal Aid scheme, but this does not currently cover industrial tribunal work, should your case reach that stage.

I've just been told I will need dialysis in under six months. Should I tell my employer and work colleagues? If so, how and when?

It will be difficult not to tell them. Even if everything goes well, you will need some time off work when you start dialysis. Most people on dialysis can expect two hospital admissions a year (of about 5–10 days). They will notice these too.

How and when you tell your employer is important. If you are in full employment when you are first diagnosed with kidney failure, telling people is likely to cause you anxiety. It may be helpful to delay a few weeks, after considering the following points.

(i) Before telling your employer, talk to your GP, renal social worker or other members of your renal team, about what it is realistic to aim for in terms of employment. Think about whether you would like to continue to work full-time, or explore possibilities to reduce to part-time or possibly to take early retirement if this is an option for you.

(ii) However well you trust your colleagues, it is probably not sensible to tell them about your condition before telling your employer. Most employers will appreciate hearing this type of information first hand and respond better.

(iii) If you work for a large company, there may be a company policy on long-term sickness – check your company handbook and contract before meeting your employer so you know the facts.

(iv) You may want to ask a representative from the personnel or human resources department to be present when you talk to your manager about your situation.

(v) It may be helpful if there is someone your employer can contact about your condition. Ask your renal social worker, GP, or another member of the renal team. They will be able to answer questions about the likely impact of your condition on your ability to do your job. These may cover how much time you are likely to need for appointments and sick leave, and other practical concerns your employer may have. They will also be able to explain how some forms of treatment are particularly well suited to those in employment.

(vi) Your employer may wish to send you for a medical assessment by a doctor selected by the company. This is a reasonable request and there is usually no reason to decline. Any costs should be borne by the company.

I've just started APD and see no reason why my disease should affect my work (in a warehouse). However, I get the impression my bosses want to 'ease me out' of the firm. I have worked for them for 12 years, and never had a day off until now, so I'm very angry. What are my rights?

Employment and disability law are complex areas. If you feel you are being treated unfairly by your employer or are in dispute, you should seek advice from a solicitor specialising in employment law. However, the following information may also be useful.

(i) If you want to continue working, your diagnosis alone is not a reason for terminating your contract. If you believe you can continue to carry out your duties effectively, you should be given the opportunity to demonstrate this.

(ii) You are legally entitled to 'reasonable' time off for medical appointments. However, the amount of time you take off sick is likely to be of concern to your employer if they feel it is affecting your ability to do your job. In some cases, an employer might stop accepting your sick certificates, or put in writing that the time you take off due to your condition is affecting your ability to carry out your duties. If this happens to you, seek advice from your union representative or the Citizens Advice Bureau.

(iii) Your employer may make you a financial offer to leave your job (eg severance payment, early retirement or similar). Don't make any quick decisions, however attractive the offer may seem – always take legal advice before accepting.

(iv) If you are registered disabled, you will receive protection under the Disability Act in addition to the usual rights under employment law. Your GP will advise you if you are likely to qualify.

When I have to go into hospital, I feel guilty about the pressure this puts on my work colleagues who have to cover for me. What can you suggest?

Unfortunately you may find there are periods when all you seem to do is spend time in hospital, so there is no easy answer to this problem. The treatment for kidney failure is complex and can have all sorts of complications, which can come on very suddenly. Part of the problem for your colleagues may be the unpredictable nature of your admissions, rather than the number or length of them. Your renal unit may have information sheets they could read – or give them this book!

Remember that if the positions were reversed, you would probably be willing to help a colleague in similar difficulties.

My job is physically demanding. Sometimes I feel exhausted and struggle to do a full day's work. My colleagues seem to think that now I have regular haemodialysis I should be fit and well again. They don't understand how I feel. What can I do?

Most people have little knowledge of kidney failure and its effects. They may think that with dialysis you are 100% fit again, and that once you have a transplant, you are cured. Maybe you need to explain to them that dialysis is by no means perfect, and provides only 5% of the function of two normal kidneys. This is not enough to make you feel well all the time.

Is it at all possible for you to get less physical work? Your employers may be able to help by offering you a different role. Job Centres also have specialist staff to advise on work for people with health problems.

Do I have to tell people at work that I'm having dialysis?

There is no need to tell anyone at work, unless your condition affects your ability to do your job. However, it is probably better to let them know, because there will be times when you have to miss work due to clinic appointments, or short admissions to hospital. If you are applying for a new job, you may be asked about your health record. If this the case and you do not tell employers the truth, you would have no protection in the event of dismissal, since your contract would not be valid.

My partner is 39 and is about to start haemodialysis. I am 35 and do not work. We have three children and are very dependent on his income. He would like to carry on working and have home haemodialysis. Is this possible?

There are many advantages to home haemodialysis. Some patients even feel it offers a quality of life second only to transplantation. You can plan your treatment according to your convenience, making changes to suit your life. There will be no travelling or waiting time to take into account. He will be able to have dialysis for four, or even five, hours, whereas few hospitals are able to offer more than three hours to many patients these days owing to lack of resources. You will not incur any costs, because the hospital pays for everything that is needed.

The 'best' sort of treatment is very much a matter of individual preference. Some patients prefer CAPD or APD (see pages 96–98) to home haemodialysis. Others want to keep all evidence of their renal failure out of the home, so prefer hospital haemodialysis. If your unit has evening dialysis sessions, your partner might be able to dialyse after work. He will probably need to do this for a while in any case, while home treatment is being arranged.

It sounds as though home haemodialysis could suit you and your partner very well. However, home haemodialysis is a joint undertaking, since he will need a dialysis helper – preferably you. The helper is only needed at the start and finish of treatment, so during the hours in between, you will only need to be within earshot, to help with any problems that might occur. Your unit will have installed a telephone in his treatment room, so calls can be made to nurses or technicians in the unit to sort out any difficulties. It is also advisable to have a back-up helper, perhaps another family member, so you do not feel you are always 'on duty'.

Talk to your renal unit to confirm they have a home training programme, and let them know you are interested. Some units may not consider people for home haemodialysis if they are likely to get a transplant in the near future, since the cost of setting up home treatment would be wasted if a transplant became available straightaway. If there is no immediate plan for a transplant, your unit will assess whether your partner would be a suitable candidate for home treatment, and discuss with you both what is involved.

Setting up home haemodialysis treatment usually takes 4–6 weeks. Your partner will need reliable, permanent access such as a fistula (see pages 113–116). Once he is stable on hospital treatment, the two of you should be able to learn how to perform his dialysis at home. A room in your home will have to accommodate the equipment but most houses don't need any structural changes. You both need to be thoroughly confident before you dialyse at home. A reduction in council tax is available if you have to have a specific room for dialysis.

Relationships, family and friends

I have just been diagnosed with kidney failure. How can I tell my family and friends? I am going to be such a burden on them.

When you first tell family and friends about your illness, they will be shocked. Anyone close to you is likely to experience the same initial reactions as you (see page 218). However, if they have been concerned about your health, they will probably be relieved that the cause of your symptoms has been determined.

When discussing your condition with those close to you, try to make sure you communicate the following to them.

(i) Kidney failure can be treated but not cured. However, treatment – especially a transplant – will enable you to lead a full life and do many of the things you did before you were ill.

(ii) No one is to blame for kidney failure – no one should feel guilty about it.

(iii) You plan to find out as much as possible about kidney failure and take a positive approach to living with it. You hope you can count on their help and support. Offer to direct them to sources of information.

(iv) Your aim is to be positive, but inevitably there will be times when you will be down and depressed. Ask for their patience and understanding during these times.

(v) Encourage those close to you to share their feelings with you, and not hide them. You are not the only one who will feel down – they will too, and that is normal. Sometimes, it might help to have a good cry together.

(vi) There is a lot of help and support available to people with kidney failure, and to their families and carers. Invite someone close to accompany you to your appointments and meet members of the team at the renal unit, or to come with you to a meeting of your local Kidney Patients' Association (see page 270). This will give them an opportunity to ask questions of their own, and meet the people who will be playing an important part in your life.

I am a trainee mechanic, 19 years old, and have a girlfriend the same age. We hoped to get engaged, but recently, out of the blue, I became ill and had to start dialysis. Now I am on CAPD four times a day, and I'm off work. My girlfriend says she will stand by me, but what have I got to offer her now? I'm not even interested in sex any more.

You have one of the best possible assets, if you have a girlfriend willing to stand by you. Let her know how much you appreciate her. One of the problems with feeling low and tired is that you may be irritable and difficult to live with – partly because you have lost confidence in yourself and cannot see how anybody could value you. You may feel you are no longer the same person she loved before your kidney failure, but it is your circumstances that have changed, not you.

If your job training is 'on hold' due to the treatment, talk to your renal unit. It is possible another form of treatment such as APD or haemodialysis would enable you to carry on, so you get your qualifications. Your lack of interest in sex may be partly psychological, and partly due to your kidney problem, so discuss this with your doctor. There may be counselling available which could help both of you.

It must be difficult to see light at the end of the tunnel, but the chances are that by the age of 21 or 22, you will have a successful transplant. You should then be able to plan for the future and think about marriage and starting a family.

I am on CAPD, and do four exchanges a day at home. I am concerned about the impact of my illness on my three young children, especially during the school holidays. I am always ill, always doing dialysis in my 'special room'. Where can I turn to for advice?

Children may appear not to notice or be affected by your kidney failure. On the other hand, they may be worrying excessively and showing it in different ways (eg, bad behaviour, poor sleep, struggling at school). Some good advice is 'talk and share'. Let their teachers know you are a kidney patient. Tell the children about your disease and why you have to keep going to the hospital. You might want to take them with you. As you are on PD, you could make the time while you are doing an exchange their 'special time' – for reading with them or talking about their day in school. Older children may be able to do a school project about your disease. If you are in the local Kidney Patients' Association take your kids along to meetings and other events. Get them interested in raising money for kidney patients.

I'm the father of two boys aged four and six. They keep asking questions about my treatment. Surely they are too young to understand about my kidney failure? I'm on hospital haemodialysis.

They may be too young to understand all about your treatment, but they are certainly not too young to realise that something is wrong. Children often fear the worst if they sense that one parent is ill, and the other is worried. Even young children are afraid that an ill parent is going to die. It is far better to explain what is happening in simple terms, and invite questions. Ask if you can bring them to see you dialysing in the unit, so that your trips to hospital are not shrouded in mystery. Children of this age are very matter-of-fact, and usually accept the dialysis machine without turning a hair. Let them feel useful. Even a four-year-old can press the mute button to cancel an alarm on the machine.

Our eight-year-old son seemed to have accepted my need for dialysis, but now he is falling behind at school and seems to be bullying other children. What should I do?

Hopefully his teachers know about your difficulties, and can help him to express any worries he has. It is possible that life at home centres around illness and treatment and he is feeling jealous of the attention you receive. You probably have less time than other parents to do things with him, such as taking an interest in his school work. Bullies are usually those who are feeling insecure, so it would be a good thing if he could be reassured of your love, at the same time as receiving your firm views on his bad behaviour.

I am on haemodialysis, and can't play with my grand-children any more, as I get so tired. What can I do?

This may be more difficult for you than it is for them. Children adapt more easily than we do. Your pride is at stake, as is your fear of growing old. Can you change your activities, spending more time reading or playing board games? Here is your chance to learn more about computers – allow them to teach you.

I am on CAPD. My daughter is taking her GCSE exams next year. She is a bright girl, but recently she often claims to be ill with tummy upsets and headaches. Our doctor cannot find anything wrong with her. We are concerned because she is missing a lot of school. Could this be something to do with my illness?

If she is anxious about you, about her school work or the possibility of becoming ill herself, her symptoms could be indirectly connected to your kidney failure. She has probably heard a great deal of talk about illness and hospitals for several years now. If she has any worries, she is likely to show them in the language she knows best – the language of being ill. Rather than taking her to the doctor again and again, reinforcing a sense of physical illness, try to find out whether she has any particular worries. She may need more attention and encouragement to get involved in interests and activities.

I feel inadequate as I cannot work and do not have the energy to control my teenage children as I should. Where can I turn for help?

As all parents know, having teenagers in the house can be stressful. They challenge, argue, and can also be very expensive. Their school may be able to help; it is always worth letting their teachers know you are having problems. Your local Social Services may also be able to advise, or refer you to the Education Welfare Officer. Most of all don't lose heart and do try to keep lines of communication open and remain friends. Teenagers do grow up in time.

**I know what you mean when you say family and friends
don't understand. How can I contact other patients with
the same problem as myself? I had a transplant last
January which only lasted a week. I've only been
diagnosed with kidney failure for two years. It was very
sudden with no warning at all. I still feel quite numb and
very bitter about the whole thing.**

If your renal unit has a local Kidney Patients' Association, this is
probably the easiest way to meet people in a similar position. If
you have access to the Internet (at home, at work, at your local
library or an Internet café) there are a number of websites where
you can chat to others over the web. See Appendix 3 for website
addresses.

**Since my wife became ill, a lot of our friends have stopped
visiting. How can we show them that kidney failure is not
catching and that we need visitors?**

This is a common complaint among people who have
experienced any sort of chronic illness. 'Friends' seem to be able
to sustain a relationship if an illness is short-lived, and even rally
round for a while, but most of them cannot keep it up. But don't
be too hard on those who drift away. Often they are embarrassed
and feel helpless because they cannot make things better. They
literally don't know what to say – which makes it uncomfortable
for them to be around those who are ill.

It may not be worth trying to get such friends back, but there is
no harm in trying. Why not invite them round for drinks, or tea.
Better still, if you feel up to it, invite them to join you on a trip
somewhere, perhaps to the cinema or the pub. This will show
them you can still enjoy normal life. If that doesn't work, you
should be looking for other friends, perhaps via a club or
patients' association.

Ask yourself too, whether you are partly to blame. People
coping with illness in the family often expect others to do most of
the work in keeping relationships going. Those 'others' may be
unsure what to do and may think you would actually prefer to be

left alone to manage. They may have made a tentative offer of help, and have been told, 'No, no, we are fine'. If you get better at accepting offers of help, others mostly feel useful and valued, and may come back for more!

I would be interested to hear how partners of kidney patients cope. I am trying to support my husband by reading lots – probably too much and scaring myself! I encourage him to exercise and watch our diet. But I worry so much about the future and how he will get on.

The partners of kidney patients are often unsung heroes and heroines, but may feel taken for granted by the patient and the hospital staff. It is a good thing for you to know as much as possible about the illness and treatment as it applies to your husband. But since every patient is different, a lot of the information and possible future problems will not apply; and may, as you say, cause unnecessary worries.

The most important support a spouse can give is to show that their partner is still valued and loved for his or her own sake, regardless of the illness. Encouragement to lead as normal a life as possible is also a great help. Over-protection and fussing can limit and irritate the patient. If you spend all your time monitoring diet, medication, and watching for adverse effects, you will exhaust yourself and drive your partner mad – remember, there is quite a bit of leeway and flexibility in the treatment. Missing an occasional tablet, or even an occasional PD exchange, having a short haemodialysis session, or breaking the diet from time to time, will not result in disaster.

Patients usually feel guilty towards their partners due to the illness, so it is actually helpful for both of you to maintain your own interests and social life. If you have a local Kidney Patients' Association, you could join it and meet other spouses. It is wonderful to find out there is someone in your area with similar feelings, who understands your experiences.

I'm gay and I care for my partner with kidney failure. He has AIDS and I am HIV positive. I go to a carers' group but I don't really feel welcome and I get the feeling they think my relationship is not as special as theirs. I want help from people who really understand.

There is a lot of ignorance and prejudice around, so you are probably right about the attitude of the other carers, which would make it hard for you (or them) to feel comfortable when discussing your relationship. On the other hand, some of the feelings may be an oversensitive or defensive reaction on your part. Either way, you are certainly right that someone who has no first hand experience of HIV and AIDS can't really understand what you are going through. For this reason you really need to get in touch with an HIV and AIDS support group in your area. Hospital social workers should have contact numbers, or you could get in touch with the Terrence Higgins Trust (see Appendix 2) which can advise you on local groups.

I don't mind looking after my Dad, who is on haemodialysis. But I am angry with my sister, who never comes to visit. I've given up my job to care for Dad, but my sister doesn't contribute anything financially and she never phones. What can I do about this?

Sadly this is a common situation, and it is not surprising it makes you angry. Perhaps your sister cannot cope with her own feelings about illness, and is frightened of contact with your father. It may be worth letting her know you need a break, and suggesting she takes over the job for a week or two while you get away somewhere. You could add that if she is unable to do this, she could contribute to the cost of a live-in carer during your absence.

Sex and fertility

I am a man in my 50s who had lost all interest in sex over the last two years. Now I have just been told I have kidney failure, and patients often have sexual problems. I am so relieved! I thought there was something wrong with me!

You are quite right – there is nothing wrong with 'you'. You have not lost your masculinity, you are just suffering from an illness that, for physical reasons, may make you lose interest in sex.

My husband, a dialysis patient, had not made love to me for two years, and I was getting desperate with frustration. Finally we saw a counsellor, who asked him if he ever had an erection nowadays. He said that sometimes in the early mornings he did for a short time, but I was always fast asleep then and he didn't like to bother me. I wish he had told me! A few days later we were able to make love.

An erection occurs when extra blood enters the penis, and is not allowed to leave. Your husband's kidney failure has probably been making it difficult for him to get an erection. It is often in the early morning that hormone levels (the chemical substances that help with an erection) are highest and drug levels lowest (some drugs, especially blood pressure tablets, have side effects that make it difficult to get an erection), and the possibility of lovemaking is most likely. It often helps if a couple chat about their problems as they may find there may be a way to solve the problem. For example, you did not mind at all being woken up early in the morning to make love.

I was convinced my husband had found somebody else, because he was avoiding having sex with me. I tried buying pretty nighties and even sexy underwear, but he wouldn't even have a cuddle anymore, let alone make love. I didn't realise it could be due to his kidney failure. Now, I can cope with his loss of interest, but I wish he would still have a hug and a kiss.

Many men who are unable to get an erection are afraid of affectionate cuddling, in case the woman expects them to go further and make love. Physical contact is also a reminder that that they are unable to make love 'properly', which might make them think they are not 'a real man' anymore. This a great pity, because everybody needs the reassurance of affectionate physical contact from time to time.

You might well benefit from some relationship counselling. An organisation like Relate may be particularly helpful – you will find the telephone number for your nearest branch in your local telephone directory.

I have been married for 15 years, and love my wife very much. We had a good sex life up until last year when I became ill with kidney failure. I don't seem to get aroused by her anymore, though I find other women attractive and fantasise about sex with other women. Is that normal?

This is a common reaction in men who have a very loving and caring partner. The role of your partner often changes when you are ill. She becomes more of a mother than a lover, which can affect the way you feel about her and act towards her sexually, since you may need to feel dominant and 'masculine' to become aroused. It is far easier to feel like this in a fantasy relationship. If you are able to talk to your wife about this it may be helpful. If you are not making love at present, your wife may also be fantasising about sex. That would be normal too. If you cannot talk together, you could try seeking help from a renal unit (or Relate) counsellor to rediscover your sexual relationship.

I've always prided myself on . . . you know . . . 'getting it up'. I'm now on dialysis, and I can still get it up but, I can't keep it up. What's going on? My girlfriend will leave me for someone else unless you can sort this out.

This problem is called impotence, and occurs in up to 90% of male dialysis patients. Even though kidney failure causes impotence, there may be other factors involved. For example, both diabetes and a poor blood supply to the penis (which can be linked to renovascular disease) can contribute. The treatment depends on what has caused the problem in your case. Your doctor will want to make sure you are not underdialysed, so that your general condition improves. If you are anaemic, you should be given EPO and/or iron supplements. Making the anaemia better gives you more energy, and can help with your sexual problems.

It is also a good idea to check all the medicines you are taking, since some tablets can affect a man's ability to have an erection. If this is the case an alternative tablet can often be found. Your doctor may also check your hormone levels, especially your testosterone level, and give you supplements if necessary. However, a low testosterone is unlikely to be the whole cause of the problem. You may be asked about your relationship and your feelings, since these may be making matters worse.

If none of these is effective, you will be offered alternative treatments, which might help. None of these treatments can increase the desire for sex, but all can make having sex possible by giving you an erection.

One method is to use a special tubular device (an ErecAid or vacuum device, see Figure 14 overleaf) that helps the penis to fill with blood. The blood is then prevented from escaping by placing a ring around the base of the penis. The device is then removed, leaving you with a good erection. After ejaculation, the ring is removed.

There is also a drug treatment called MUSE (Medicated Urethral System for Erection). This involves the insertion of a small tablet into the end of the penis, using an applicator. When the tablet dissolves, the drug (aprostadil) increases the blood supply to the penis and produces an erection. The drawback with this method is that the erection can continue long after love-making has ended, and there is some risk of discomfort.

Sildenafil (Viagra) is a drug taken by mouth, which can produce an erection – if you are doing things that normally lead to an erection. In other words, it is not an aphrodisiac that immediately makes you sexy and gives you an erection. It does not last longer than you want it to, which is an advantage. Not everyone can take this drug safely, so you should consult your doctor. People who have had heart attacks, or suffer from angina or have very high blood pressure, may be advised not to take sildenafil.

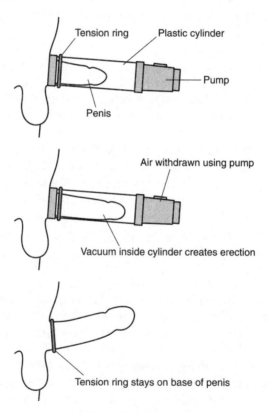

Figure 14 An ErecAid

Is Viagra suitable for women?

Viagra is not licensed for use in women. It has also not been tried in female kidney patients. So, it should not be used by any woman at present. However, there have been some research studies into the use of this drug in women, and it has been found to have some effect on creating juices in the vagina and making you feel more like having sex. There have been recent reports of successful pregnancies in women (without kidney failure) taking Viagra, who were previously unable to have babies. Viagra appears to improve the blood supply to the whole genital area, and may cause the lining of the womb to thicken due to better nourishment from the bloodstream. It is likely there will be further developments in this type of treatment for sexual problems in women.

If I have a transplant will my erections return to normal?

Yes, as a general rule sexual function, including the ability to get an erection, improves after a transplant. It is not always the case, because in some men the problem is caused by other factors, such as relationship problems or diabetes, which are not cured by transplantation.

I am very tired and worn out after my haemodialysis session and don't really feel like lovemaking. My partner feels I have gone off him and doesn't seem to understand that I do love him and just don't feel like making love. What can I do?

Patients on dialysis often feel very tired, especially following a session on the machine. Other causes of loss of sex drive can be depression, anaemia, or a change in roles between you and your partner. It is important your partner knows he is still valued. Try to show him that you love him. You could also try planning something romantic, like buying a bottle of champagne, on the days when you are not tired.

Discuss the problem with your doctor when you visit the clinic, because it may be that your medication is not helping the situation. You may also be feeling bad about yourself. Some patients have problems with the way they look (especially those on dialysis, because of either the catheter or fistula) and no longer feel desirable. This can lead to avoiding sex with their partner. If the problem continues, ask for referral to a counsellor.

I feel a real freak since having a PD catheter in my tummy. I don't like my husband to see me undressed any more because I feel so unattractive. I always think people in the street must be looking at me and thinking I look odd.

Dialysis patients often get very self-conscious about the way they look. If it isn't the catheter, it's a fistula or tunnelled line, which also make patients feel unattractive. From what you say, you probably realise it is you, not your husband or other people, who thinks the catheter is ugly. Perhaps, because you have lost confidence in yourself, you don't feel like making love any more. Maybe your husband thinks you no longer find him attractive. You may not have a lot of inclination or energy to spare for him at present. But the sooner you start thinking about his feelings rather than yours, the sooner you will be able to forget about being self-conscious. Talk to your husband about your feelings – he will probably be very relieved you still want him to find you attractive. If you can reassure each other about this, and express affection for each other, you will be well on the way to regaining your confidence.

Will anyone fancy me anymore?

This is a common, and understandable, worry for patients on dialysis. Coming to terms with kidney failure is not easy. The truth is, however, that you are the same person with the same lovable characteristics that you had before your kidneys failed. There are practical problems in living with someone who needs dialysis or a transplant, but these can be overcome if you find the right partner to share your life. In spite of the problems, you are likely to find somebody who fancies you! It is however important you are happy with yourself, because those who believe they are attractive often behave in an attractive way, and encourage possible relationships.

I am a 35-year-old woman and in a fulfilling relationship, but recently I am finding sex painful. What should I do?

Sex should be a pleasurable experience and not painful. You may have a problem with a lack of lubrication (producing juices in the vagina). You could try having more foreplay. If this does not produce adequate lubrication, try a water-based lubricant (like KY jelly) which is available from your local chemist. If lovemaking continues to be painful, ask your GP to check there are no other problems, such as an infection of the vagina (for example, thrush), or of the womb. These should be treated with appropriate antibiotic or antifungal medicine.

I am on CAPD. Can I have sex while I have a dialysis bag in?

Yes, it is perfectly safe to have sex while you have the dialysis fluid inside. But you can drain the dialysis fluid out if it makes you feel more comfortable. Try out some different positions and make sure your catheter is secure as it will make you feel more at ease and prevent any dragging on your line.

Can I have sex while connected to the APD machine?

Yes, it is possible to have sex while on the machine. Sometimes you may trigger an alarm if you lie on the tube but give it a go. If you have problems, disconnect while you are making love. You may have to try out different positions and remember to secure your line.

I have noticed that since my kidneys failed, I have developed breasts (I am a man!) It is very embarrassing, and I have to keep my shirt on . . . what can I do about this?

It is common for men to develop breast tissue (gynaecomastia) when their kidneys fail. It can be due to the medicines you are taking or hormone disturbances. The level of the hormone prolactin is often raised in men with kidney failure, causing the development of breast tissue. If you are very upset by this symptom, discuss it with your doctor, who may refer you to an endocrinologist (hormone expert) who can prescribe drugs that may help. If tablets do not help, you may require surgery.

I am a kidney patient and have been with my partner for some time. She can't seem to get pregnant . . . could it be me?

Yes, it is possible. The toxins that build up when they are not removed by the kidneys may interfere with the way your body makes sperm. This causes a reduction in the number of sperm and also their ability to swim. If you are concerned, ask your GP if you can have a sperm count done. You may also be referred to a fertility clinic.

If you have had a transplant, it is likely your sperm count will return to normal once toxins are cleared from the body and hormone levels restored.

I have been on haemodialysis for the last five months and continuing to have periods on a regular basis. I have met a man and want to have a sexual relationship with him. I have heard that women on dialysis can't get pregnant. Do I need to take the Pill?

You *can* get pregnant! Even if you are having irregular periods or no periods at all, there is still a risk of getting pregnant. So, if this is the case, you should also use some form of contraception.

If you want to take the contraceptive pill, you should contact your unit and make an appointment to discuss it. The Pill is best avoided if you have high blood pressure or clotting problems. You can discuss other methods of contraception, such as the coil (intra-uterine device) or condoms, with your doctor.

You should also be practising 'safe sex' to reduce the likelihood of getting AIDS and other sexually transmitted diseases, by getting your partner to wear a condom.

My periods stopped soon after I started dialysis. Will they start again after I have a transplant?

Most women find their periods start again as their hormone levels return to normal after a transplant, and there is better clearance of the toxins from the body. Oestradiol is one of the hormones controlling your periods, and this is usually restored to normal after a transplant, resulting in a return of normal ovulation (egg production in the ovaries) and periods.

I'm on PD and am desperate to have a baby. Is pregnancy advisable? Where would it fit inside a tummy full of dialysis fluid? Would it be better if I was on haemodialysis?

Successful pregnancy means producing a healthy baby without harming you. This is rarely possible either with advanced kidney failure (say a creatinine of over 300 micromoles/litre of blood) or for women on dialysis. Pregnancy is not advisable, because there is a high risk to you and the baby. However, if you decide to attempt a pregnancy, it should be carefully planned with your doctor. If you were to go ahead and try for a baby, you should first be aware that you might not be able to get pregnant. Kidney failure and dialysis reduce fertility. If you do get pregnant, you will have a high risk of miscarriage. It may also make your blood pressure dangerously high.

The chance of a successful pregnancy in a dialysis patient was very poor in the past. But this has improved over the past few years. The most important aspect of management is making sure you are getting enough dialysis. For a haemodialysis patient that can mean having dialysis every day to keep the urea level in the blood below 17 mmol/litre before and after dialysis.

It is possible to continue on PD while pregnant, as the fluid is in the peritoneal cavity and not in your uterus (womb) where the baby will grow. They are quite separate. The abdomen is able to stretch a great deal, and can accommodate both the growing baby and the PD fluid. However, as the pregnancy progresses, the amount of dialysis fluid may need to be reduced and you may need to do more exchanges. Some sessions of haemodialysis may also be needed to keep the blood chemistry as good as possible.

There is no clear evidence that haemodialysis is better than PD, although some women swap to haemodialysis as they find it uncomfortable to carry both fluid and baby. Usually babies born to women who need dialysis are born early and are smaller than average.

Overall, it is better to wait until you have had a transplant, both for your sake and for the baby's. But although the risks of being pregnant while you are on dialysis are quite high, it is ultimately your decision. It is the job of the hospital team to support you in whatever decision you make.

I've have been told I have 20% of my kidney function left and I have a creatinine of around 400 micromoles per litre. I will probably need to start dialysis within six months. Will it harm my kidneys to get pregnant?

Yes, becoming pregnant may well mean you need to start dialysis sooner than expected. You should discuss this with your doctor as you may need dialysis while you are pregnant. There are many things you may wish to consider such as your age and how easy it will be for you to get a transplant in the future. If it is possible for you to wait until you have a successful transplant, it would probably be better for both you and the baby.

I'm an Asian woman aged 25 years, and I've got a rare disease called lupus. I've been told that I have got 75% kidney function (my creatinine is 150 micromoles/litre) and that I will probably have to start dialysis within the next five years. My husband's mother wants me to get pregnant. So do I (sort of) but my husband does not want me to come to any harm. What should I do?

It is much more likely you could have a successful pregnancy now, than if you wait for a few years. But if you are at all unsure about whether you want to have a family, you should talk to your husband first. The decision to start a family is yours and his, and nothing to do with either your parents or his.

I am a pregnant kidney patient on haemodialysis. Can I deliver my baby normally?

A normal delivery is possible, but if the mother is on dialysis, the baby frequently has to be delivered early by caesarean section. This is usually because the mother is suffering from a condition called pre-eclampsia, which occurs in the later stages of pregnancy and is more common in women with kidney problems. Pre-eclampsia causes a dangerous rise in blood pressure, making early delivery essential.

I'm 25 years old and have a good transplant, with a stable creatinine of around 80 micromoles/litre. I've just found out I'm pregnant. Even though I'm overjoyed, I'm worried about the baby, and my transplant. What should I do next?

You should make an appointment to see your consultant and get advice about what to do, and if your medications will be a risk to your unborn baby. Pregnancies in women with transplants are often successful. There is a small increased risk of an episode of acute rejection (this happens in about 10% of patients) and about 15% of women have a miscarriage within the first three months. This compares to about 10% of women without kidney failure.

Who will look after me in pregnancy?

You will be under the care of both the kidney and maternity teams. They will work together with your general practitioner and midwife. It is important to monitor your kidney function (at least monthly if you are not yet on dialysis) and blood pressure during your pregnancy.

I have a transplant, and I am expecting my first child. Can I breastfeed while on cyclosporin?

Cyclosporin is passed on through breast milk, so you would be advised not to breastfeed.

Complementary therapies

I'm a kidney patient. Might complementary medicine have anything to offer me?

In recent years, some types of complementary medicine have become widely accepted by conventional medical practitioners. Acupuncture and homeopathy are now available in some NHS hospitals. Chiropractice and osteopathy are also receiving recognition from doctors in the treatment of conditions such as back pain. Hypnosis is accepted as useful, especially in dental practice for pain relief, reducing bleeding following extractions, and for some irrational fears including needle phobia. Few doctors would now claim that complementary treatments have nothing to contribute – particularly if they are used as their name suggests, not as an alternative to conventional treatment.

Not all the effects are understood. Many doctors accept that acupuncture works, but have little idea why. Some may have a psychological component, but any therapy that makes the patient feel better without serious side effects can only be a good thing. The value of a positive and optimistic mental attitude cannot be overstated. There is evidence that the immune system, which fights infections and guards against cancers, can be more effective if the patient has a positive state of mind – and can become less efficient as a result of stress, grief and low mood states.

Complementary therapies have always recognised the value of a holistic approach to illness – treating the whole person, mind and body, rather than a set of physical symptoms.

No 'respectable' complementary treatment would claim to cure ESRF, but some therapies are beneficial in improving the morale, quality of life and sense of well-being of those with kidney failure. Symptoms such as poor sleep, pain and restlessness on dialysis, needle phobias, itching, lack of energy and tension headaches can often be improved by complementary therapies, including 'talking therapies' like counselling. But it is important to use these treatments carefully and wisely.

I have kidney failure and am receiving dialysis treatment, but I am not sure I really need it. Dialysis does not make me feel any better. Couldn't I try herbal remedies or homeopathy?

If you had to start dialysis before you began to feel really ill, you may wonder whether the treatment is necessary. But kidney failure makes you unable to get rid of substances that are normally expelled by the kidneys in the urine. Even if you are passing adequate amounts of urine, it may not contain the toxins and excess chemicals that need to be removed. This is why kidney patients need lower doses of many conventional drugs. For the same reason, you should not try any herbal remedies for your kidneys or any other problem, without first talking to your doctor. Herbal remedies can be very powerful substances, which might be toxic for a kidney patient. Homeopathic remedies are less risky, because they are usually given in extremely small amounts.

If you believe that you do not need dialysis treatment, and are passing good volumes of urine, talk to your doctor who will examine your blood test results. These will show exactly how much work your kidneys are doing.

I am a dialysis patient. Massage and aromatherapy make me feel better and more relaxed. Are these treatments suitable for kidney patients?

Any treatment of this sort, that makes you feel relaxed and increases well-being, is certainly good for you. Massage helps the circulation and is comforting in itself. Any form of relaxation reduces stress and helps to lower your blood pressure. The aromatic plant oils used in aromatherapy can affect the emotional state, encouraging pleasant thoughts and sensations and producing a beneficial effect.

I have been on dialysis for a long time and have painful renal bone disease. Would it help to see an osteopath or chiropractor?

Kidney failure causes weakening of the bones due to loss of calcium. Dialysis patients may also develop deposits of a protein called amyloid, which can cause painful joints, especially in the wrists and shoulders. If you were to see an osteopath or chiropractor, it would be very important that they knew about your kidney failure, and had access to your X-rays. Manipulation of damaged or weakened joints may not be advisable. Ask your doctor as both osteopathy and chiropractic can help in the relief of pain. If you have badly damaged hip or knee joints, you might need joint replacements. Painful wrists are often improved by a fairly minor operation called a carpal tunnel release.

8
Coping with kidney failure

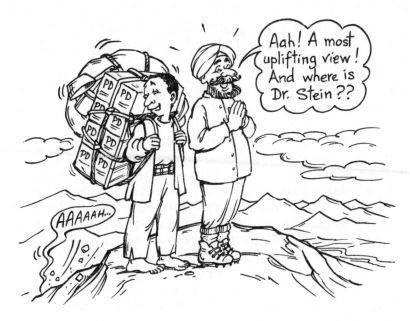

When all is said and done, kidney failure is not pleasant. As the disease progresses, difficulties are likely to increase. This chapter looks at some of the ways you can cope with the tougher aspects of life with kidney failure.

Psychological problems associated with kidney failure

I started dialysis six weeks ago. I thought I was doing so well, but suddenly it has all got on top of me and I'm really depressed. Is this how it's going to be from now on?

Starting dialysis is like facing any other crisis. Most of us can rise to the occasion, be brave and determined for a short time, but it's hard to go on without letting our real feelings show. Sooner or later there is a bad day when it all seems to overwhelm you. At first it is a new challenge to have dialysis, and you are relieved to feel better physically. As time goes on, the novelty wears off, and you become aware that although there are some improvements, dialysis cannot make you feel 100%. There are good days and bad days, and you cannot rely on feeling really well. It begins to dawn on you that this situation is going to go on, and on – unless you are suitable for a transplant.

At this stage, your courage has been running on 'empty' for a while, and you suddenly have no more resilience left. Your feelings are absolutely normal so don't be afraid to let them out. Crying is actually better for you than anger, and better too for those close to you. Talk to them if you can, and explain how you feel. It is frightening to feel out of control, but you will come through it. If you go on feeling very low, let your unit know, and they will arrange somebody for you to talk to.

Kidney failure and its treatment affect everything in your life, and the lives of those close to you. Relationships and roles may change. You may find you are irritable, especially with those you love best. Like any other big adjustment in life, it is usually accompanied by some symptoms of stress or distress. You should not feel you are weak or different if you go through periods of anxiety, anger, or depression. You may also have feelings of bitterness, helplessness and loss of control over your life. These are natural reactions to what is happening. Some patients say that following diagnosis of kidney failure, they experience feelings similar to a bereavement – losing somebody you loved dearly. At first there may be shock, numbness or disbelief, then sharp grief, alternating with anger. This slowly eases towards acceptance, but it can take time.

Most patients work through the negative feelings and return to some sort of positive attitude. There may be situations that trigger a recurrence of uncomfortable feelings from time to time. Let your unit staff know if you want to talk about how you feel, because talking often helps more than anything else.

When I was told I had kidney failure and would need dialysis in future, I thought 'no problem'. I wasn't going to die, so I told myself it would make no difference to my life and put it out of my mind. Now, my doctor says I am 'in denial' and suggests I see a counsellor! Why? I feel OK and I still don't need dialysis.

It's very natural to react in this way. In many ways you are right, things are not all that bad, so why dwell on the fact you will need dialysis? But some people carry this attitude to extremes. They decide not to take their medication, such as blood pressure tablets, or not to bother to attend clinic appointments.

As long as you look after your long-term future health by taking advice on drugs and diet, and going to your check-ups, a bit of 'denial' may be the best way to handle the situation. People at the renal unit are always a bit worried if someone thinks being on dialysis 'will make no difference'. It does make a difference, but not necessarily a big one, especially at the start.

The treatment takes time, and you may need to think hard about how best to fit it into family life, your job and all the things you like doing. If you plan ahead, finding out for example which type of dialysis will suit you best, you will be prepared for the future, and will probably adjust to treatment better when the time comes. It's natural to put something out of your mind if you are so frightened that you can't really face it. This is why your doctor thought you might need help. If you can face it, learn a bit more about what will happen. This way, you will have a head start when you need dialysis.

How can I keep occupied while on the haemodialysis machine? It seems to take up so much of my life, and I feel guilty that I am not doing anything.

One of the problems of haemodialysis is that it is hard to concentrate during treatment. There can be lots of interruptions due to machine alarms, and noises around you. This may make it hard to enjoy a good book or do office work or the household accounts. It is better to find something that can easily be picked up and put down, like puzzle books, crosswords or magazines. Sewing and knitting may be possible, depending on your access. This is not confined to women. One of the most contented patients we know is a hefty six-foot postman, who produces the most exquisite embroidery!

Watching television can be relaxing, though you may get bored with the game shows. If you have a video, you could record the evening programmes to watch during the day. There's no need to feel guilty – after all, most people spend two hours or more each day watching the television. Tapes of music and books are popular, and some patients use relaxation tapes and learn to make the times pass therapeutically. You could try learning a foreign language from tapes, and then plan a holiday abroad. You could be even more ambitious and start an Open University degree.

I feel as though I can't bear the thought of the future on dialysis, and it's making me very depressed. What can you suggest for coping with this?

Many patients feel as you do when told they will need dialysis. Once treatment starts, there is usually a 'honeymoon period', when you feel relief that the treatment is not as bad as you feared and dialysis makes you feel physically better. Almost all patients then go through a further period of depression after a short period on dialysis. Usually this is a temporary stage – part of coming to terms with the loss and limitations dialysis involves. Knowing it is a normal reaction which should pass may help you. Although knowing things will get better is not the same as feeling hope for the future. It is a hard adjustment to make, and there will be times when you feel nobody can possibly understand what you are going through. Depression is often linked to feeling you have no control over your life and you are at the mercy of circumstances. It may be helpful to realise you are now more in control of what happens to you than you were before starting dialysis. Your health and well-being are now very much your responsibility.

It can be a good thing to plan small targets, to show yourself you can achieve something in spite of what has happened. It need not be a big thing – something like doing a small repair that has been hanging about for ages, writing a couple of overdue letters, making a phone call you have been putting off. Once you feel a bit more confident, it is a good thing to start investing in the future, instead of being wrapped up in a daily struggle with the present. It is up to you how you do this, but the important thing is to fix your mind on the future, and the fact that life goes on. You can give yourself little rewards for getting things done, and enjoy feeling you are making progress.

Your problem with depression may be more severe, for example if you experience any of the following:

(i) persistent feelings of your own worthlessness;

(ii) a conviction that your family would be better off without you, or nobody would miss you if you were dead;

(iii) crying spells, day after day;

(iv) problems getting to sleep, or early morning waking.

If these symptoms are present, you need professional help. Talk to your GP or your renal consultant. A course of antidepressant medication might be a good thing, although talking to someone understanding might be what is needed.

I've been on haemodialysis for two years now. The renal unit staff are kind, but so busy they never have time to talk. I try to keep cheerful when I come for treatment, but at home I'm quite different. Everything and everybody gets on my nerves – my husband, who is wonderful, and our children. They deserve better. What is wrong with me?

You are bound to have some bad feelings, for example anger and frustration at being on dialysis and not being able to do all that other wives and mothers do. If you put on a brave face when you are at the hospital, those feelings will come out somewhere else and affect those who are most important to you. Perhaps you should tell your nurse what you really feel, and ask if you can talk to someone. Most renal units have a social worker or trained counsellor who will help you to express these feelings in a place where they can do no harm, and help you find ways of coping with the anger.

My sister, who is 23 years old, and started dialysis six months ago, gets very tired and can't seem to 'pull herself together'. She has known for years this was coming. Surely she could make more of an effort?

Many dialysis patients feel extremely tired and lethargic all the time (partly due to anaemia, see page 50). Some will be feeling very low as well – especially as they know they will need dialysis treatment or a transplant for the rest of their lives. There is no cure. They can feel their life has been turned upside down, so it can be very difficult to 'pull themselves together'. Some renal patients need the help of a psychiatrist, psychologist or counsellor to help them to cope.

My husband, a haemodialysis patient, is getting very depressed – especially since the doctors said he couldn't have a transplant as he is too old (he is 70). What is the best way to cope with his depression while he is ill?

It must be very upsetting for your husband to feel he is trapped on dialysis for the rest of his life, and even more so if he feels there is discrimination on account of his age. Your doctor was less than tactful, if age was given as the reason for the decision. There may be other factors that affected your doctor's opinion. Usually the decision to transplant or not depends more on the patient's general health than their age – there are some 40 and 50-year-olds who would be advised against having a major operation under general anaesthetic. It is a question of balancing the risks and benefits.

As far as life expectancy is concerned, your husband is likely to live just as long on dialysis as with a transplant, as are most renal patients, whatever their age. It therefore seems to be a question of helping him to come to terms with his dialysis. It may be he needs to go through a period of anger and adjustment to the loss of his previous way of life. Most patients experience depression at some time in the first year of dialysis treatment – some earlier, some later. He may start to show the symptoms of clinical depression (an inability to sleep, tearfulness and feelings of worthlessness). If he does, you could discuss with his doctor whether anti-depressant medication might help. It is more likely he needs to express his feelings about the situation. Then, with your help and encouragement, he may begin to enjoy some of the things he liked before all this happened.

Professionals

My doctor is always late for clinics and keeps us all waiting. He can't be at emergencies all the time. We are all fed up. What can we do?

We all know that doctors are busy and overworked, but if this is happening regularly, the organisation of the clinics needs investigating. The knock-on effect of late appointments, combined with transport problems and difficulties with home and work responsibilities, can become intolerable. So too can the irritation of sitting for hours in waiting areas.

There are formal complaints procedures in every hospital, which you can access by requesting the forms to make a complaint. But it may be better to start by writing a letter to the Consultant in charge of the unit, with a copy to the Manager of the renal unit, politely explaining what is happening. If you get no satisfactory commitment to try to improve matters, along with an apology for the situation, you should write to your local Community Health Council which handles complaints and grievances. They help and advise patients and relatives who wish to complain about any aspect of their treatment under the NHS. Their number should be in the telephone book.

As carer for my father, who is on haemodialysis, I should be kept fully informed about my father's illness. But my father's doctor says she is bound by confidentiality and can't discuss any details with me. Is this true?

Yes, this is true. However, you are absolutely right that it would make it easier for you to care for your father if you knew about his condition. You need to talk to your father and ask if he would be willing to tell your doctor, formally in writing if necessary, that he has no objection to your knowing details about his condition. He might also be happy for you to attend his clinic visits, so you can hear for yourself what is said. Two heads are often better than one at remembering what advice has been given. If, on the other hand, your father does not wish information to be given to you, I'm afraid there is no way the doctor can compromise the trust of her relationship with her patient by disclosing details without permission.

My doctor never seems to have time to go through all my problems. Would it help if I sent him a list?

Clinic doctors are always under some pressure to keep the clinic running to time. It may be that to go through all your problems is too much to expect in the time available. It is also possible that a nurse, dietitian or social worker would better handle some of your concerns. If you were to send or bring a list, the doctor could quickly tell you which problems he or she was best able to help with, and refer you to other team members to deal with the rest. You can also request an extra long session with your consultant outside normal clinic hours. Ask next time you go to the hospital.

I find the doctor who is treating my sister very rude and abrasive. Who can I talk to about this problem?

If your sister is also unhappy with her doctor, perhaps you and she should start by discussing it with the renal social worker who can act as her advocate. It is perfectly reasonable to ask to be transferred to a different doctor, on the grounds of a personality clash. You or she should write politely to the head of the unit she attends, with her request. Not everyone can get on, and when someone has a chronic illness such as kidney failure, it is essential there is a good relationship between patient and doctor. They are going to see a lot of each other over a long period. Obviously, if a number of people make the same request concerning the same doctor, management will realise there is a problem, and perhaps give guidance, a reprimand or suggest the doctor takes a job elsewhere. If there are no other consultants at your sister's renal unit, she can ask to be transferred to another renal unit if this is what she wants.

My doctor gave me the wrong dose (ten times the normal one) of Alfacalcidol. It put my calcium up and made me very ill. Even though I want to make an official complaint about him (especially as he didn't have the decency to say sorry) I'm frightened by what he can do to me. What should I do?

It is always frightening to risk angering someone who you depend upon for your health. But you really have to act, not only for yourself but also for other patients – and even for the doctor himself. If he is under strain or overtired due to problems at home or at work, causing him to make errors, it needs to be investigated. If it had been another drug, a single dose ten times too large could have been fatal, so it is a very serious matter. Amazingly, it sounds as if a simple 'sorry' might have allowed this doctor a second chance. In this case, perhaps you should visit the Hospital General Office and ask about registering an official complaint with the hospital's Complaints Department. You may also like to contact your local Community Health Council, who will give you practical help with lodging a complaint. Do not worry about being labelled because you 'blew the whistle'. Nothing will happen to put your care at risk. There is bound to be another doctor in your renal unit who could see you instead.

Doctors are aware these days that they must maintain standards. Even if this means reporting a colleague for bad practice, they are now obliged to do so. Remember, if a registered gas fitter set the pressure in your central heating boiler ten times too high and caused an accident, he would lose his Corgi accreditation – at least until he had gone through retraining! Why should doctors be any different?

How can I find out who my consultant is? No one seems to know.

Most units allocate each patient to a particular consultant nephrologist (kidney specialist) in the unit. This does not, of course, mean you will always see the same person every time you visit the clinic. If you ask one of the nurses, they should tell you the name of your consultant. Normally the consultant is named on your admission wristband when you are an in-patient. The consultant's name may also be on a board by your bed.

In some hospitals, patients are given a consultant depending on the type of treatment they have. For example, all PD patients are looked after by one consultant, transplant patients by another and haemodialysis patients by another. You may therefore change consultant when you change from one treatment to another. There are some hospitals where patients are not allocated to one specific doctor. This can be very frustrating for patients.

How can I contact my consultant? His secretary never seems to pass on messages.

It is not practical for consultants to be contacted all the time for day-to-day queries. The doctors called registrars usually handle these. Most secretaries try to protect their bosses from interruptions, but you should certainly be able to make an appointment to see your consultant if you have a particular problem. Telephone his secretary and ask for an appointment. Or better still, write to him explaining what you want to discuss so he can get together the relevant information to answer your queries. Most consultants have bleeps that work over long distances, and you can ask the hospital switchboard to get them to call you back.

I'm on PD. I've heard that in most renal units, community PD nurses visit regularly. Although my PD nurse is very supportive, she says it is not the unit's policy to visit patients in their homes. Can this be true?

Yes, I'm afraid it can. Not all renal units have community PD nurses, although there has been some research showing that visits at home prevent expensive hospital admissions. This means they are cost effective, as well as good for patients. If you want to change your unit's policy, get together with other patients and your local Kidney Patients' Association, and let the consultant in charge know how you feel. You may not get change at once. But keep at it, and eventually you will get the service you need.

What does the renal social worker do?

There is considerable variation in the social work service in renal units in different parts of the country. Some hospitals now employ care managers, who are social workers specialising in the assessment of patients for home care services on discharge from hospital. These social workers may or may not be willing to help with problems such as claiming benefits, counselling and advice on problems other than care needs. Most renal units cover a large area, involving more than one county. A social worker or care manager is employed by a specific county or metropolitan area, and is generally unable to visit patients in their own homes, unless they live within their area. Most hospital care managers are also discouraged from working with outpatients, since their responsibility is to those in hospital. Outpatients are usually referred to their community social worker, who may have little knowledge of the problems a renal patient may face.

This situation is not at all satisfactory. It has resulted in some renal units employing their own specialist renal social worker, paid by the unit or a charity such as the BPKA rather than Social Services. If you have such a social worker, he or she should be able to offer a full range of services to patients. This may include liaison with community workers, help with benefits and welfare rights, advocacy, counselling for individuals and couples and advice on all non-medical aspects of care.

What is a care manager?

A care manager is a social worker whose particular job is to assess and arrange provision of care in your own home. Once care is in place, your care manager should monitor what is happening, and respond to any changes in your needs.

Social services are going to provide a home help, because my husband has kidney failure. What sort of jobs will the home help do? (I am 78 years old and not well myself.)

There is some variation in policy in different parts of the country, so this answer may not apply fully to your area.

Social Services provide home care, supplied either by their own or agency carers. These carers are trained to help with personal care (for example, helping a patient to get up, go to the toilet, wash and dress, as well as preparation of meals where needed). If your husband has been assessed as needing help with personal care, the carer will usually do other jobs for you, such as a bit of cleaning, washing or shopping. But if your husband needs no personal care, and all you want is somebody to do cleaning and washing, you will usually be offered the names of local agencies which will provide domestic help. It is likely you will have to pay the full charge for this service. The charges for personal care are adjusted to your means and savings, and may be very small.

Are there any specialist nurses who might be able to help my husband? He's a blind diabetic on haemodialysis and has terrible leg ulcers. I can't lift him any more.

District nurses from your GP surgery are able to dress ulcers. You should ask your GP if you would like them to visit regularly to do his dressings. It sounds as though you have many other problems. If your husband's mobility is severely impaired, you need to ask for an assessment by the community occupational therapist. Your district nurse or social worker can arrange the necessary referral. There are pieces of equipment and a number of aids and adaptations which may make it easier for him to move around. For example, he may not be able to get out of bed or up from a chair without your help, due to the height of the furniture. If the bed or chair is raised, he may find it much easier and you will not risk damaging your back.

If your husband is registered blind or partially sighted, he may be eligible for a number of additional benefits. Speak to your social worker about this.

What does the community dialysis nurse do?

Unfortunately, not all renal units provide a community dialysis nurse. His or her main role is to act as a link between the home and hospital, so reducing the need for frequent hospital visits. Community nurses can take blood samples, blood pressure, check your fluid balance and give general help and advice on medical matters.

They also provide a good form of contact with your hospital consultant.

Carers

**I am a full time carer for my husband, who is on haemo-
dialysis and very disabled. He cannot do anything for
himself. But I married him 'in sickness and in health'.
I feel guilty when I say 'I feel trapped'. Can you help?**

If you are a carer for someone with kidney failure, you may feel
everything is geared towards help and support for the patient and
your needs take second place. But you mustn't feel guilty about
thinking about yourself and your own needs. Caring for someone
can be rewarding, but there may also be times when it is difficult,
and you resent the role. This is entirely natural, but it is important
to recognise your well-being is also a priority, and not to feel
guilty about thinking of your own needs. There is help and advice
available to make sure you look after yourself too.

- The renal unit staff and your GP will recognise the
  importance of your role and will be happy to discuss your
  difficulties (either practical or emotional), and advise you on
  ways of dealing with them. They may be able to put you in
  touch with local agencies to help with the practical aspects
  of the care you provide, or with someone who can help with
  counselling for any emotional difficulties you may be having.

- Don't put your own life on hold. Try to keep up with some of
  the hobbies or activities you enjoyed before, and keep in
  touch with your own friends. If the person you are caring for
  has difficulty recognising the importance of this for you, or
  resents time you spend away from them, ask for help in
  explaining it to them from the renal unit or your GP.

- Check out the local voluntary groups. Organisations such as
  the **Carers' National Association** and **Crossroads Care**
  exist to help and support carers. They may be able to
  arrange to give you a break on a regular or occasional basis,
  depending on the level of care you provide.

- Sometimes it can be helpful to talk to others 'in the same boat'. There are various support groups available for carers, where you can meet up with other carers and discuss common problems and experiences. Ask whether your GP or local Kidney Patients' Association can recommend a group in your area. The Carers' National Association and Crossroads Care may also run a local support group, or put you in touch with one.

What about me? As the carer for a PD patient (my elderly mother) I feel that no one is looking out for me. There are only the two of us in the house.

Looking after anybody full time is a draining experience, especially when the dependent person is an elderly parent. The roles are the reverse of those in childhood. However good and loving the relationship, there are uncomfortable emotions and conflicting feelings. There is bound to be resentment, guilt and a sense of feeling trapped. It is important you maintain a separate life of your own, as well as caring for your mother. There will come a time when she dies, and you will be left alone. You should not feel guilty about spending time away from her. If you have any interests you can pursue for an afternoon or an evening a week, arrange for a respite carer to take over. Talk to the renal social worker, a local carers' association or your Citizens Advice Bureau about agencies that could provide somebody to help.

Under the Carers and Recognition of Services Act 1995, you are entitled to an assessment of your needs as a carer in your own right. If you discuss the matter with your GP, it may be possible to arrange occasional or regular respite care for your mother in a residential or nursing home. Many homes now have PD trained staff if your mother needs help with exchanges. This would enable you to get away on holiday, or just to have peace and quiet at home. Your mother may be resistant to the idea, but will probably benefit as much as you from the break.

My father is on haemodialysis. Is it normal to get angry and lose my temper with him? Are all carers supposed to be saints?

People who are ill are not necessarily easy to live with. Sometimes, they can be self-centred, angry, irritable and demanding. Other times they may be pathetic, self-pitying and over-helpless. You may get very little thanks for all you are doing. Worst of all, they are often able to cheer up and be all sweetness and light when other people are around, and only show their real feelings to those closest to them – the ones they can really trust. This is a sort of compliment, but one you would probably prefer to do without. It is normal to feel guilty if you lose your temper with 'someone who is ill, poor thing'. But the truth of the matter is that those who are ill need to learn they cannot be persistently unpleasant or demanding to their nearest and dearest, without affecting them.

It is treating your father as less than a person if you make endless allowances. You must stand up for yourself, gently but firmly. Also, make sure you are maintaining some sort of life of your own, which should give you more patience and tolerance at home.

My husband with kidney failure is able to do less and less, partly because I am doing too much for him. Should I back off?

You seem to have answered your own question by saying you are 'doing too much' for him. This is not good for either of you. He will feel more and more useless and dependent, and you will get overtired and resentful, especially if you think he could do more. It is however, quite difficult to get somebody to do more for themselves if they have got into the role of 'invalid' and are used to being waited on. Your husband may complain or get upset if you ask him to do things for himself. But as long as you are not unreasonable, and coax him encouragingly, you and he may well find he can do far more than he believes.

Are there any training courses for people caring for someone with kidney failure? My wife who is 72 years old, is about to start dialysis.

Ask in your unit about education. Some hospitals run a programme of training for patients and carers. Relatives are welcome at educational sessions. If you need to train as a home haemodialysis helper, you will be taught the procedures in hospital for several weeks before returning home with the patient to dialyse. If you need to perform CAPD exchanges or help with APD, you will also receive full tuition in hospital.

If you attend clinic visits with your wife, you can talk to the dietitian and medical staff about diet and drug regimes, and ask any questions you want. In fact, it would be a good idea to accompany her to clinic, just in case important information is forgotten.

My husband has recently been diagnosed as having kidney failure. I am in my early 70s and still very fit. We have no children. How long am I likely to be able to carry on caring for him? If I die what will happen?

If you are fit and well, there is no reason why you cannot look after your husband for many years to come. If at any stage it became difficult, either because you were not so well, or needed help with heavy care like lifting, or perhaps just because you needed a break, there are services available to help. Ask your social worker about care at home, and whether you would have to pay for this. It would depend on your savings. This would cover his personal care needs such as help with washing, dressing and toileting. Your district nurse would be able to help with any nursing care required. Realistically, if your husband is as old as you are, or older, you are likely to outlive him. This would be true whether or not he had kidney failure. However, should he outlive you, he could either continue to be cared for at home with help from social services and district nurses or, if he preferred, he could enter a residential or nursing home.

I've been caring for my wife, who is on haemodialysis. But now I have had a stroke. We want to go on caring for each other, but I'm afraid. How can I care for her if I'm disabled?

From the practical point of view, you may need help with caring for each other, either now or in the future. This could mean getting some home care from Social Services, or might eventually mean entering sheltered housing, a residential or a nursing home together. Most homes cater for couples, and let them live as independently as they are able. Discuss this with your renal social worker, or local Social Services Department.

The most important thing to understand is that you will still be caring for each other. Caring is not just cooking, shopping, washing and dressing someone. Caring is showing interest, sympathy and affection; letting someone express their feelings, whether good or bad, and not withdrawing from them. Caring can be sitting peacefully in silence with somebody, knowing there is understanding and support between you. This sort of care is far more important than practical help, which can, in fact, be given by just about anybody. You are probably the only person in the world who can supply the real emotional care your wife needs.

How to get help, practical and financial

What is respite care and how do I get it? My husband, a haemodialysis patient, is becoming very frail and I feel I cannot leave him.

Respite care can be arranged through your GP or social worker, depending on your husband's needs and your own finances. It is a short stay in a cottage hospital, nursing home or residential home, to enable you to take a break away from home, or even to have a rest at home without the pressure of responsibilities. Many carers find it hard to take a break, even when it is offered. So it is sometimes better to go and stay with a relative, or take a proper holiday. You may be tempted, otherwise, to visit your husband every day while he is away! It is sometimes possible to arrange a regular break, perhaps one week in six, to enable you to carry on with care at home. Discuss this with your GP or social worker. The cost will be met by the NHS if your husband needs hospital care. But if he goes into a residential home, the charge will be means tested by social services.

Respite care may be provided in your own home, enabling you to get away for a break. In addition, some carers benefit from a sitting service – a few hours off to enable them to get out to shop or attend a club or other activity. Voluntary organisations, such as Age Concern, or Crossroads may be able to provide this service. You may also want to find out if there is a day centre locally which your husband could attend. Ask your GP or social worker.

How can I get practical help at home? I am 67 years old and live alone.

Contact your renal Social Worker and ask for a referral to the Home Care Department of your local Social Services Department.

If you live alone, you may be concerned that as your kidney failure progresses you will need support to carry on living at home. This may range from help with your shopping to having someone help with your personal care.

I am on PD, and set a room aside for my treatment. Can I get a reduction in council tax?

Yes, you can apply for a 'disability reduction' of your council tax. What usually happens is that your banding limit is reduced to the next lower level. Contact your local Council Tax office.

Can I get help with the cost of travel to hospital for dialysis and check-ups?

It depends on your current financial situation, and what benefits you are receiving. If you have income support, income-based jobseekers allowance, working families tax credit or disabled persons tax credit, you can be refunded for your travel costs by the hospital – once you have shown proof of entitlement (eg your pension book). If you have already paid you may be able to apply for a social fund grant to cover the costs. You will need to apply to the DSS within three months of buying your ticket. If you are not on any of the above benefits but have a low weekly income and your savings are under £8000, you can apply for a certificate of full or partial exemption of charges. A few units allow a small mileage rate for those who drive themselves in for dialysis treatment. Ask whether your unit is one of these.

Would a carer who travels with a renal patient also get reimbursed?

If you are to claim travel costs for a carer, your doctor must sign a declaration that you need an escort. This could be for a number of reasons. Children obviously qualify. Somebody who is blind, or suffers from learning disabilities, who cannot speak the language, or cannot understand what is said at the clinic visit (eg because they have had a stroke) would also qualify for an escort. Ask your social worker.

I need to use a wheelchair – how can I get one?

Under the NHS, wheelchairs are supplied and maintained free of charge to a disabled person whose need is likely to be permanent. If the need is temporary, a wheelchair can be supplied on loan by the British Red Cross. If your need is likely to be long-term, ask for a referral to your local Occupational Therapy (OT) Department or Mobility Centre for assessment. Your GP or OT section of Social Services can complete the referral for you.

I've heard you can get a car with Mobility Allowance. Can you tell me more?

If you have been awarded higher rate Mobility Allowance (part of Attendance Allowance or Disability Living Allowance) for life or for a period of at least two years, you can take advantage of the

Motability Scheme. This allows you to hire or hire purchase a car or electric wheelchair by asking the DSS to pay your mobility allowance directly to the Motability Scheme. If you qualify for a Motability vehicle, you can choose to hire or buy an electric scooter instead of a car.

The vehicle will be supplied by a participating garage or dealer. Many dealerships now offer Motability vehicles. You should receive details of the scheme when you are sent notification of the award of DLA Mobility component.

If you receive the higher rate of DLA Mobility Allowance, you are exempt from road fund tax (VED). You should automatically receive an exemption form from the DSS.

My husband, who is on haemodialysis, has had to leave his job as he is so ill all the time. Will his pension rights be affected?

The situation regarding your husband's occupational pension will need to be clarified with his employers. As far as the State Pension is concerned, this is dependent on his National Insurance contributions. He will receive a National Insurance credit for as long as he is sending sick notes from his doctor to the local Benefits Office.

I'm approaching dialysis. My doctor keeps putting me on more and more tablets but I can't afford them. Are there any other ways of paying? Can I get free prescriptions when I'm on dialysis?

This is a complicated issue, and 'the rules' are open to interpretation. It is well covered on the NKF website (see Appendix 3).

There are four main ways of getting tablets.

   (i) **Pay conventionally** – ie, pay for items one by one. Most GPs will give you prescriptions for three months' worth of tablets at a time. Even so, this can be very expensive if you are on a lot of tablets.

(ii) **Pay by 'Prepayment Certificate' (season ticket).** If
this is your preferred option, you will need an application
form (FP95) from your hospital pharmacy. Currently, you
will only make a saving on a four month season ticket if
you need more than five items in that time. Over thirteen
items during a year will give you a saving on an annual
season ticket. Once you have one, you can put as many
items on them as you like within the period covered.
But whenever prescription charges go up in price, season
tickets do as well.

(iii) **Automatic exemption.** If you are under 16 years old
(16–18 years if you are in full time education), 60 years or
over, pregnant, a War Veteran, or receive any of a variety
of benefits from the Government, you will not need to pay
for your prescriptions. You may need to prove that one of
these states apply. Booklet HC11 (also from your hospital
pharmacy) explains this in more detail.

(iv) **Medical exemption.** You need another form – this time
it's called a FP92A. If you have certain long term diseases
or treatments, you can also get prescriptions free. These
include epilepsy, diabetes, thyroid disease, physical
disabilities and a 'permanent fistula'. So, if you get one of
these forms, if your doctor is willing to state you have a
fistula (many kidney doctors will consider a PD catheter
a type of fistula), you can get free prescriptions when you
start dialysis. After a transplant, the rules are a little more
open to interpretation, but most kidney doctors will be
willing to help wherever they can.

So, to answer your question . . . you may be able to get free
prescriptions when you start dialysis. Before that, you may have
to pay. If you do, a season ticket may be the cheaper option.

I have been turned down for the disability benefit I applied for. How can I appeal? Even though I've got a good transplant, I can't walk.

You are entitled to appeal against the decision to turn you down. You simply have to write to the Disability Benefits Centre whose address will be on the letter you have received, and say you want to appeal. There is usually a time limit of 30 days. If you are too late, you can reapply, but this means filling in the forms all over again. If it is less than three months since you were refused, you can ask for a review of the decision, sending any supporting letters from your doctor or social worker that can be arranged. You can get help with appeals from the Citizens Advice Bureau and from your renal social worker.

Where can I get advice about benefits and grants?

The array of benefits can be confusing and daunting, as can the forms you need to fill in to claim them. You can get advice from the Department of Work and Pensions (see Appendix 2) but, if you have financial concerns, it is probably better to discuss your situation first with your renal social worker.

The Citizens Advice Bureau can also provide advice on benefits and help in completing the required paperwork. In many areas there is a Welfare Rights Advice Centre, able to give independent advice, help in completing forms and assistance with appeals. If you cannot find one in the telephone book, ask your Citizens Advice Bureau if they know of a centre near you.

Some charities have grants available for patients and their carers. Examples of the types of help that may be given are assistance with the cost of a holiday, fuel bills, home improvements or alterations needed as a result of illness or disability. You may apply to more than one charity for the same reason, and your application will be treated in confidence. Charities who have awarded grants for kidney patients include the British Kidney Patient Association and the National Kidney Research Fund.

I'm on haemodialysis now. If I have a transplant, will I lose my benefits?

When you have a transplant, all your benefits will be reviewed. Many transplant patients have their disability benefits, such as DLA or Attendance Allowance, changed following a review. In some cases, the patient is so much fitter that he or she no longer qualifies for personal care or mobility payments. In others, there is still a need for these benefits, and they are renewed. Incapacity Benefit is usually continued for a few months, because the frequent clinic visits make it impossible to return to work.

I have had to give up work to look after my husband. Are there any benefits I can claim?

If you have given up work to care for your husband, you will be entitled to Invalid Care Allowance (ICA), provided you are below retirement age. You are able to get ICA even if you still work part time (less than 16 hours per week). This benefit affects other means tested benefits such as Income Support and any payment to your husband for you as a dependent (for example he might be getting an increase for you in his Incapacity Benefit). If this is the case, you will not gain financially from getting Invalid Care Allowance. It is however worth having, because as long as you receive ICA, you will get a National Insurance Credit to protect your own future pension rights. Get a leaflet about the benefit from your local DSS office.

I retired early to care for my sister, who has kidney failure. Can I get grants or financial help from anywhere other than the Benefits Agency?

Most Kidney Patients' Associations can give a limited sum towards emergencies, but not regular payments to make up shortfalls in income. Local Kidney Patient Associations and the BKPA may be willing to help finance holidays and often have their own facilities to offer. Other associations may make specific grants, and charities such as Rotary Clubs or occupational charities may also be willing to help (see Appendix 2 and your local telephone directory).

Where can I find out about benefits and financial help for carers?

If you think you need financial assistance, or want to find out if you would be eligible to receive benefits, it may be helpful to talk to someone who 'knows the system' first. If the renal unit has a renal social worker, he or she will be happy to advise you. Or you could ask your GP to put you in contact with a community social worker. They will be able to advise you on which benefits you could apply for, and help you with filling in the forms.

The Citizens Advice Bureau can advise on benefits and help with the paperwork. The Carers' National Association will also be able to provide information and advice on benefits for carers.

If your house has been adapted in any way to make it easier for the person you are caring for to manage, you may be entitled to a reduction in Council Tax. Contact your local council Tax Office and request the forms to apply.

What is community care and how do I get it? I'm on haemodialysis.

Under the Community Care Act 1990, anyone who wants help with personal care while living at home is entitled to ask for an assessment by the Social Services Department of their Local Authority. The help you need may be very little, for example, delivery of meals because you find it hard to cook a main meal for yourself. However, a great deal of help may be needed. You may need help to wash, dress and get to the toilet. It may be necessary for somebody to visit you three times a day to deal with your needs and check that all is well. If you think you need help, contact your local Social Services Department whose number should be in your telephone book. Explain you want to be assessed for community care. Your hospital social worker may be able to refer you if you do not feel able to do it for yourself.

What is a 'needs assessment' for community care?

Once you have asked for assessment of your needs, a social worker called a Care Manager will visit you and ask a number of questions about your condition and the help you need. Following this assessment, you will be asked about your financial position, to decide whether you will have to pay for any or all of the care. Your savings will be taken into account. You will also be asked if you receive DLA personal care component, or Attendance Allowance. If you get either of these benefits, you may have to contribute part of this money towards your care. If you receive Income Support and have very few savings, you will not have to pay for care.

What can I do if I don't agree with the needs assessment or with the amount of help offered to my Mum, a PD patient?

You are fully entitled to ask for a review of the assessment of your mother's needs. Social Services have leaflets covering what to do if you disagree with any decision, and setting out the procedure for making a complaint if you do not think you have been fairly treated. Ask your hospital social worker what you should do if you are in doubt.

I've recently started PD. Where can I get advice on legal and financial matters?

If you do not have a solicitor, try the Citizens Advice Bureau, who may be able to answer your questions. If they cannot do so, they will give you a list of solicitors who will offer advice under the legal aid scheme, or for a reasonable charge. The Citizens Advice Bureau are also able to advise on financial matters including benefits.

My widowed mother, who has kidney failure, has always been a well-organised person and she doesn't like me to interfere in her financial affairs. However, she is finding it hard to cope and I don't know how to help. What can you suggest?

If you are elderly and ill, it is sensible to grant an Enduring Power of Attorney to somebody you trust. It is impossible to know when you may be suddenly incapacitated and need somebody else to handle your finances. If you prefer, more than one person can be granted a Power of Attorney for you (eg if you have two children, you could appoint both of them, so either could act for you, or you could specify that both should agree and sign on each occasion). Why don't you ask your mother to do this?

Power of Attorney is arranged by a solicitor, and enables an Attorney (eg you) to handle a person's affairs. It has to be arranged with the consent of the person concerned (in this case, your mother), who also signs the document. Your mother should be legally fit to consent with full understanding of the implications, at the time of signing. You can then act for her in any way you see fit – sign documents, cheques, pay bills, transfer money in and out of bank accounts – in fact make any financial decisions that she herself could make.

This means you have to be fully trusted by the person concerned. If your mother is mentally fit to manage her affairs, and does not wish to give you Power of Attorney, there is nothing you can do. If she becomes mentally unfit, which is a medical decision, you would need to apply to the Court of Protection. Your solicitor will give you details.

My husband, who has kidney failure, has always looked after our money and paid all the bills. I want to take this burden off him now he is ill. How can I, or our daughter, take over the finances?

Discuss granting an Enduring Power of Attorney with your husband. He may be willing to allow you or your daughter (or both of you) to act for him.

My father is on haemodialysis and he is very ill, and confused off and on. Can he still make a will or sign an Enduring Power of Attorney?

Yes, provided he is mentally capable *at the time of signing* the will or Power of Attorney.

I have recently been diagnosed with kidney failure and I want to make a will. Are there any special things I should think about?

Every adult should make a will, be they young or old, fit or suffering from an illness. Nobody knows what the next day will bring.

See your solicitor and explain you have a kidney condition, which could have implications for your future. The solicitor should be able to advise on any special provisions advisable due to your illness, such as minimising estate duties, and may also suggest you give a friend or relative Power of Attorney to handle your affairs if necessary.

How does my newly diagnosed kidney failure affect my insurance policies? Will I be able to get a mortgage?

Policies taken out before you developed kidney failure are not affected, only new policies. Providing you are generally fit, apart from kidney failure, you should be able to get a mortgage. The National Kidney Federation has details of brokers who can find 'kidney-friendly' insurance companies and mortgage providers.

Practical concerns

I am overwhelmed with boxes of PD fluid – they are stacked everywhere. I am afraid I am going to trip over them and fall. Is there any help available with storage facilities?

Under the Chronically Sick and Disabled Persons' Act (1970) your Local Authority has a duty to make arrangements for provision of services, including any adaptations needed due to your medical condition, for your 'greater safety, comfort or convenience'. If you can demonstrate that the boxes of fluid are a potential risk to your ability to move around your home, the Local Authority can address this by supplying a garden shed, for example, or adapting an existing space. Most Local Authorities need persuading that your needs come under the act, arguing that, as part of your medical treatment, it is the Health Authority's responsibility to fund storage for dialysis supplies. In some units, storage facilities are provided out of the home dialysis budget. It is worth persisting. Contact your renal social worker, or Social Services Department (OT section) for an assessment.

I have kidney failure and am on dialysis. Is there any reason why I shouldn't carry on driving?

Treated kidney failure should not mean you cannot drive. There is a long list of conditions that the DVLA ask you to report, including major illness such as kidney failure, epilepsy, a recent heart attack or stroke. This is because, if you were to have an accident, you could have problems with your insurance company if you had not declared some relevant health problem to them and to DVLA. Talk to your doctor about exactly what you should notify the DVLA about, and write to The Drivers' Medical Unit, Morriston, Swansea, SA99 1TU. They will send you a form to complete and may contact your doctor for further evidence of your ability to drive.

Since I have been on PD, I have been told I cannot take a bath or go swimming. Is this true?

The advice for bathing and swimming is different. If you are on PD, it is probably better to shower, although a shallow bath that does not soak the exit site is perfectly possible. Unit policies vary on this point, so ask your PD nurse's advice. It may be possible to provide waterproof dressings if you would like to take a bath. It is certainly more relaxing to have a long hot bath and it is not surprising that you miss it.

If you are on a low income, you may be able to get financial help towards installing a shower. You may also benefit from some bathing aids, such as a grab rail to help you get in or out, or a bath board you can sit on while you swing your legs over the side of the bath. Talk to your community occupational therapist or renal social worker about these adaptations.

Swimming is a good form of exercise, and quite possible for dialysis patients if they are careful. Talk to your PD nurse before you go. You may be asked to wear a waterproof dressing while you swim, and do an exchange and clean your exit site when you come out of the pool. You should avoid swimming in lakes or rivers.

I'm 82 years old and on PD. I'm having problems dressing myself. How can I make things easier?

If you need help with getting yourself ready for the day – whether washing, shaving, dressing or preparing breakfast – it is possible to arrange for a home carer to call every day. This needs to be arranged with your local Social Services Department. Ask your social worker or the Citizens Advice Bureau for a referral to the Home Care Department. If you don't want or need a carer to come in, you could get advice from a community occupational therapist (OT). Your district nurse will put you in touch with the OT Department. Most dressing problems involve the bottom half of the body, ie pants, trousers, shoes and socks. The OT can advise on the easiest way to manage dressing. There are gadgets to help put on socks and long shoe horns to put on slip-on shoes.

You may be able to manage elastic-waist jogging pants more easily than trousers with zips, buttons, belt or braces.

Although my mother has fairly substantial savings, she doesn't own her own home. She gets the State widow's pension. Will she have to pay for home care? Or a nursing home, if it came to that?

Your mother will be assessed financially by Social Services to determine what charges she will have to pay for home care. Policy and charging vary between different local authorities, so it is impossible to give exact information. Savings are taken into account, and in most cases, those with a certain amount of savings are liable for the full cost of care. Once savings drop below a certain level there is usually a nominal charge, which also applies to those with no savings, on low incomes or on Income Support. There is always a charge for meals-on-wheels or frozen meals supplied by the local authority. (Ask your local social services or the hospital social worker for details of charges made in your area.)

Policy on payment for nursing or residential care also varies between regions. The NHS and local authorities sometimes share the cost of care, depending on whether the need is for predominantly 'social' or 'nursing' care. Ask for an assessment, to determine what kind of care she needs. Her needs will be assessed by a panel composed of Health and Social Services staff. If the local authority is responsible for your mother's care (ie her needs are for 'social care') she will be financially assessed, and will have to pay for her care until her savings drop below a certain level. If her needs are predominantly for nursing care, the cost may either be shared, or completely covered by the Health Authority.

My father is on haemodialysis and can no longer cope. He has reluctantly agreed to go to a nursing home. Will we have to sell his house? We've just had our fourth child and were looking forward to living in it?

This will depend on the type of care your father needs. If his need is for nursing care, you may not have to sell the house when he moves into a nursing home. The NHS may be responsible for payment, although this is often delayed. The reason is that Health Authorities have a limited budget for continuing care, leading to a waiting list for funding. If his care is assessed as being the responsibility of the local authority, his house will count as part of his assets, and he could be required to sell it to pay for his care. Those who have a spouse, or a family member over 60, or a relative who is disabled, already living in the house, would not be required to sell it. For more detailed information, ask your Social Services department or Citizens Advice Bureau.

If my mother has to go into a nursing home, who will do her PD exchanges? She is getting too frail and forgetful to manage them entirely herself. As I work, I cannot supervise them for her.

Many nursing homes are now employing staff who can perform PD exchanges. However, if there is no home in your area that can provide this, your unit may arrange for your mother to have haemodialysis in hospital instead.

I would really like to have a pet as I live alone and get very lonely dialysing at home. Would this be OK or is there any reason why I shouldn't get a dog or a cat?

Pets are wonderful companions, and have been shown to improve both the physical and mental health of their owners. If you are on CAPD, it would be as well to shut the dog or cat out of the room during the actual exchange, to prevent the risk of infection. It would be a good idea for you to get an animal, but remember that even a small dog needs exercise. You should be fit enough to take the dog for walks, which would be enjoyable for both of you. If you cannot do this, it could still be possible to have a pet as a companion. A neighbour might be willing to exercise a dog, or, if you have a garden, he or she could play outside for part of the day. Cats are less difficult to keep, because they are more independent and don't need exercise. They can also be left on their own for a weekend if you want to go away, or have to go into hospital for a short stay (provided you have a cat-flap). A dog would need to go to a friend or neighbour, or into kennels, if you were away. The choice is up to you.

I have heard that I could get PD infections from caged birds. Should I get rid of my budgie? I am very fond of him and would like to keep him if possible.

There are one or two reports of PD infections which seem to have come from birds, but they are very rare. It would perhaps be sensible to perform your exchanges in a different room from the budgie, especially if he is allowed to fly free. Many PD patients have caged birds which have given no problems at all, so there is no real reason to get rid of him.

I am concerned about having a pet animal. On a recent clinic visit, I was found to be in need of immediate admission to hospital. I live alone and had left my dog at home.

This is a real problem, but similar to that of a single parent, who has taken a child to school before visiting clinic, only to be admitted straight from clinic. If there is no neighbour you could trust with a key and instructions to care for the animal, you should ask the renal social worker. One of the many tasks they undertake is to rescue pets in these circumstances, arranging admission to kennels or getting help from the RSPCA.

Kidney patients who live alone need to find a trusted key-holder who can deal with this sort of emergency. Admissions can be sudden and unpredictable. It is better to make some sort of arrangement than to give up having pets, which are extremely beneficial and important companions.

Spiritual needs and dying

I want to arrange for a priest to see my father, who is in hospital with kidney failure. How can I organise this? I think he is dying.

Nearly all hospitals have a chaplaincy service, which usually provides Anglican, Non-conformist and Roman Catholic priests able to talk to patients and administer sacraments. Ask the ward sister to put you in touch. If your religion is not covered within the hospital, which is often the case with Judaism, Islam, Hinduism, Sikhism and other religions, ask the chaplaincy service to put you in touch with a priest of your own religion. The chaplains usually hold a list of religious leaders from other faiths who are able to visit patients in hospital. Also, most chaplains will visit any patient of any faith.

Why me? Having kidney failure feels like a punishment. What have I done to deserve this? Could I have avoided it? I never drank a lot or smoked too much, and I have always tried to be a good and moral person.

Kidney failure is almost always bad luck, not the result of what you have done or not done. It is not usually connected to smoking or alcohol. It must seem as if you are being unjustly punished by God, fate or whatever it is you believe in. Bad things seem to happen just as often to 'good' people as to 'bad' people. The truth is, life isn't fair. A crucial point may be that some people can find something positive in whatever nasty surprises life has up its sleeve, whereas others react only negatively and create even more sadness and misery for themselves and those around them.

I have been a dialysis patient since I was a teenager. I am now in my 40s. In the early years I coped with the situation more or less, but things have really got me down recently. When I had only myself to worry about, I could

manage, but it got worse when I married. I have wonderful support from my wife, but I can no longer bear the thought of how much my early death would hurt her. When we had a child three years ago I was thrilled, but now all I can think about is the fact that I will probably never see him grow up.

We all live with the knowledge that death can come at any time, and for kidney patients this is a real and justified fear. The truth is that none of us can tell what is going to happen. The only way to cope is to do all you can to avoid preventable causes of death such as high potassium levels, then live each day as fully as you can. Of course this is easier said than done. At a practical level, you might like to write letters for your son, which you could give to your wife: perhaps one suitable to be read to a five-year-old, one for a ten-year-old, one for a fifteen-year-old and one for when he comes of age. You can tell him so much about yourself and your experiences – also your hopes and fears for him and the assurance of your love. This would mean a lot to him, should you die before he becomes an adult.

My church has services which offer healing. Would this help me? I am a dialysis patient.

Spiritual or faith healing can certainly affect morale and well-being for the better. Patients receive a sense of warmth and support from the positive feelings and prayers of the group, and frequently report feeling better. If you would like to receive healing, it would probably be beneficial. You should not, however, feel you lack faith, or have failed in some way, if your kidney disease is not affected by healing. You should never rule out miracles, but they can come about in different ways. You may gain something you had not expected from the experience.

I have been on dialysis for many years. I suppose I kept going for my husband, but now I'm a widow. I cannot get out any longer because I need a frame. I am in constant pain and have just had enough. I would like to give up dialysis, but feel this is sinful – a sort of suicide.

Withdrawal from dialysis should never be seen as suicide, even though you would die after a few days or weeks without treatment. If it had not been for a very technical and artificial life support system, you would have died many years ago. All kidney patients are living on borrowed time. To stop dialysis is only to let nature, or destiny, take its course – to accept what would have happened naturally if you had not fought against it for so long. You do not say whether you are a religious person, but if you are, you should talk to your priest about your feelings. If you really want to withdraw from treatment, you should discuss this with your family and with your doctor. It may be you are still severely depressed by the death of your husband, or that the pain (which it may be possible to improve) is getting you down. If you still want to withdraw from treatment after discussing everything, you should receive every support from your renal unit to make your last days pain-free, peaceful and fulfilling.

My father is 93 years old, has dementia and does not know who I am. He also has Parkinson's, clots in the leg, asthma, swallowing problems, small strokes, and side effects of medications. I have to make all his decisions. He lives in an old people's home. I visit him every day. Now his kidneys are at 9%, and I have been told by his kidney specialist he will need dialysis within three months. My GP, who knows him better, says although he will need dialysis to live, he does not think it 'is appropriate' for him. Will dialysis prolong his life and improve it. Is it worth trying, and whose decision is it anyway? If we chose not to have dialysis, how much time would he have?

This is a very hard decision. There is no right answer. Dialysis may prolong his life by a small amount, but it could even shorten it too. He is only likely to live 3–6 months from now, whether he has dialysis or not. In the end, the decision is made by a combination of your GP and the hospital specialist. It is very important you let them know your views, but it will not be your decision.

Their decision will not be based on his age alone, but on a combination of his age, his other medical problems, and what an outsider would see as his poor quality of life.

My 78-year-old father has been on haemodialysis for five years. He is diabetic, blind and unable to take care of himself. His health has reached the point where my mum is unable to care for him. He is currently in hospital, awaiting discharge to a nursing home. He does not want to go to a nursing home. His only other option is to stop dialysis and go home. He has stated he wants to do this. If he chooses this, how long before he would pass away?

If your father decides not to continue dialysis, he will receive counselling and the implications of this decision will be discussed with him and your family. The medical team will support his decision as long as they are sure he is of sound mind, and is making a fully informed choice.

If he continues in his decision not to have treatment, he will be given appropriate medication to ensure he is kept comfortable and free from pain until his death. If he chooses to go home to die, the renal team will refer him to community based agencies (his GP, and district nurses) who can provide him with support and comfort.

It is a good idea for patients to let relatives and doctors know their wishes should they become unable to make the choice themselves. This could happen, for example, if they became unconscious following a stroke, or otherwise mentally unfit to decide.

It usually takes 2–4 weeks to die, after stopping dialysis; but it can be a few days or a few months. Towards the end, he will become more and more sleepy. It is not usually painful, and there is little suffering. Fluid on the lungs (pulmonary oedema) can develop, resulting in shortness of breath. Drugs (especially morphine and related drugs) can be given, if this happens.

I have decided I have had enough of life on dialysis and would like to stop treatment. Can you tell me how long I will take to die and what will it be like?

It usually takes a long time to come to the decision to stop dialysis and no doubt you have spoken to everyone involved with your care.

The time it will take you to die depends very much on the amount of kidney function you still have. If you have no kidney function and make no urine, you could die within a few days of stopping treatment. If you still make urine and have some kidney function left, you could stay alive for up to three months.

Most people who choose to stop treatment die within two to four weeks.

Once you have made your decision, it may be a good idea to put all your affairs in order. For example, you might like to make a will, plan your funeral and make sure you have said all your 'goodbyes'.

The doctors and nurses at your renal unit will do everything they can to make sure you do not suffer during your last few weeks or months. You will, however, become more and more tired and sleepy. One day you will just not wake up.

9
Research, ethics and getting involved

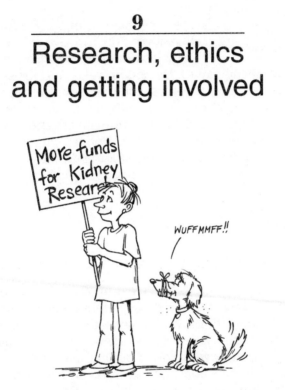

Research is an important part of improving care for patients and their families. Although this research may not help you directly, it may help people like you in the future. This chapter gives you some background on the different types of research being carried out and on the ethical issues involved.

In the UK, doctors and nurses should only use treatments that have been thoroughly researched and proven to be effective and safe. This is sometimes called 'evidence-based medicine'. Unfortunately, in the kidney world, too little good research has been done, especially in the UK. Most of the important research is being done outside the UK, especially in the USA.

So, we sometimes use treatments that have not been researched thoroughly. Next time your doctors wants to change your treatment, ask them what is the evidence that 'backs up' that change. There may be little.

For all these reasons, we feel that it is important for you to be informed about research. Ask your doctor what studies are going on in your unit. You could also stimulate research in your unit, perhaps by raising money. Do not, however, feel pressurised into taking part – there is no obligation to do so. It is important, too, to be aware that almost all research carries some risk, as it usually involves trying out new treatments. Everything is done to make these studies safe, but no guarantees can be made. There will be no penalties if you choose not to take part.

Research

What types of research into kidney failure are going on?

Every aspect of the lives and treatment of people with kidney failure is being researched by someone, somewhere. It is important to know that most kidney patients at some time will be asked to take part in a research study that may eventually benefit you, or people like you. You should consider it carefully, and discuss it with your doctor, your nurse and your family – then decide whether you want to take part. People like you make research happen, researchers only count the numbers.

The two main types of kidney research are 'laboratory-based research' and 'patient-based clinical research'.

I've been asked to give a blood sample for a laboratory-based research study. What is laboratory-based research, and should I sign a consent form?

Laboratory-based research usually takes place within hospitals that are linked to a university. It is concerned mainly with looking at how the kidneys work. Sometimes, patients are asked to take part in this kind of research. If they are, they may be asked to give a sample of blood (as you have been) or of peritoneal dialysis fluid, for example. Even for a simple blood test, you should be asked to sign a consent form if it was a blood test you wouldn't normally be having. This is the case regardless of whether or not you are being put at any risk or being asked to try a new drug or other treatment.

You may also be asked to give a sample of some of your kidney (a biopsy). This should only be taken if you were already having an operation on your kidney(s). But, some studies do involve 'extra' kidney biopsies, ie, ones that would not have ordinarily been done. This type of biopsy carries risks (see page 84). The kidney biopsy samples may be used in the laboratory to grow new kidney cells (the tiny building blocks of the body). These are then used in other studies – say, to look at the effects of new drugs before they are used on humans.

Some kidney diseases are inherited (page 12, page 74) and blood samples may be taken from patients with kidney disease and their relatives (parents, sisters, brothers, cousins) some of whom may or may not also have kidney disease.

I have been asked to take part in a study about a new type of EPO. Is this 'patient-based clinical research'?

Yes, it sounds like it. Improving the treatment of the complications of kidney failure, such as heart disease and anaemia, is an important aspect of patient-based clinical research.

The most significant advance in the treatment of people with kidney failure was the introduction of EPO injections in the early 1990s. EPO has a dramatic effect on well-being and energy levels of kidney patients because it treats the anaemia occurring as part of kidney failure. Trials are currently taking place into a new form of EPO that is taken less frequently. This new injection is called NESP, or Novel Erythropoietin Stimulating Protein and is usually given once a week or once every two weeks. The study you have been asked to take part in may concern NESP. Other researchers are looking at factors that may cause heart disease – such as cholesterol, a substance called homocystine, and smoking.

What other areas of kidney failure are being looked into at present?

Aside from research into improving treatment of complications, patient-based clinical research can be divided into the following main areas.

(i) **Preventing the progression of kidney failure.** There has been some research into ways of slowing down the damage that occurs in kidney failure. This area of research is called 'progression' – as it is trying to slow the progression (worsening) of kidney failure. This research is ongoing. The ultimate aim is to prevent people from going onto dialysis, or even getting them off it, when it has been started.

(ii) **Treating kidney failure early**. It may be better to start dialysis when the creatinine level in the blood is 300 micromoles per litre (say when the kidney function is 30%), rather than at 600 (5%) as mentioned in Chapter 3. At this stage the heart may not have sustained so much damage. In other countries, such as Holland, dialysis is often started at this 'early' stage.

(iii) **Improving methods of dialysis**. There has recently been a lot of work looking into improving the quality of dialysis. Newer techniques such as haemodiafiltration, improved dialysers and 'sodium profiling' have been put forward as ways of improving the quality of haemodialysis. The quality of peritoneal dialysis is also advancing. There is now more use of APD machines, dialysis fluids which do not use glucose, and new fluids which may help prolong the life of the peritoneal membrane.

(iv) **Improving the treatment of kidney transplant patients**. A lot of research is concerned with the development of new immunosuppressant drugs. Newer drugs may reduce the risk of rejection, and may have fewer side effects. But some of their own side effects are quite serious. So whether they are a real advantage is not known at present.

(v) **Looking at the social and psychological effects of kidney failure**. People with kidney failure are often affected by a range of social and psychological problems as a result of their disease: job losses, depression, anxiety and relationship problems. They have frequent visits to the hospital; and tightly controlled dietary, fluid and drug regimes. These have to be fitted into everyday life. The importance of providing education and support for renal patients is increasingly being recognised. Nurses and social workers have shown that well supported and educated patients do better on dialysis and live more fulfilled lives.

I'm not sure whether I want to take part in patient-based clinical research, even though I've been asked. Should I do it? Are there any benefits?

It is entirely up to you whether you take part. You should start by satisfying yourself that the study is safe. Ask to see information about it before signing the consent form and if you are still not sure don't be afraid to ask questions. However, if you are reassured on this point, we would encourage you to take part. Even though you may see no clear or immediate benefits yourself, if people like you hadn't taken small risks and become involved in patient-based research on dialysis you wouldn't have the chance of having it.

Is there national collaboration of research into kidney failure, as there is with AIDS?

Not much. Unlike AIDS, which is caused by one specific virus (HIV), kidney disease is caused by many different problems. So, different groups of doctors with different interests, research different aspects of kidney disease. Unfortunately, this means very little research has been done by large groups of kidney doctors.

The UK government does propose national research campaigns, although these often don't address renal research issues. This is because governments usually pay more attention to high profile diseases like heart disease, cancer and AIDS. If you think that more research into kidney failure should be done, write to your MP. It all helps to raise the profile of the 30,000 or so people in the UK who are on dialysis or have a transplant.

This is only part of the problem. Another problem is that kidney disease is rare – though clearly not on your unit! So, it is difficult to find the few patients in the country that have, say, your condition – which could be a rare cause of a rare disease, and therefore very rare. A comprehensive national database of kidney patients would help. The one that exists (the Renal Registry) covers less than 40% of the patients in the UK. Find out whether your unit sends data to this registry. If it doesn't, ask why.

Rivalries between different units in the UK, and between countries, also do not help. There is no one national (or international) body that co-ordinates research into kidney disease. This is also a major problem.

In the UK there is a professional society for kidney doctors, the Renal Association. This group has a committee that co-ordinates a few of the research studies taking place between more than one hospital within the UK. Unfortunately, at the time of publication there were only one or two such studies taking place. Studies like this are often submitted to the Medical Research Council (MRC) for funding. More information on the MRC can be found on their website (see Appendix 3) which also includes guidelines on patients' rights within medical research.

There are a few research centres within the UK which collaborate directly with centres in Europe and the USA. They may exchange information and technical expertise, or publish joint scientific papers.

All of this means many decisions are based on the doctor's opinion, rather than scientific evidence. Ask your consultant whether your unit is contributing to national research studies.

Which UK renal units do the most research? Will I see the results of any study I take part in?

Most renal units in the UK do some research. It is difficult to say which hospital does the most research and in many ways this is not important. The important issues are who is doing good research and who is putting it into practice. Good research goes on in many forms within a renal unit, some of which is not seen by patients. Unless you ask, you will not necessarily be told the results of the study. So . . . ask! Also, you can ask to see any publication that comes from the study.

Many UK hospitals now have expert panels to advise on the design and conduct of studies and help with funding issues. These panels are called Research and Development Committees. They are different from the hospital and regional ethics committees, which ensure that all research undertaken in the UK is done ethically.

It seems to me that not many new treatments for kidney failure ever see the light of day. Why is this?

As there are almost no drugs available that are specifically designed to treat kidney failure it may seem like nothing new ever happens. In fact new drugs for the treatment of high blood pressure, infection, kidney rejection, heart disease, bone disease and anaemia are being developed, and being used, all the time. Obviously, new treatments for aspects of kidney failure need researching. In the last 10–20 years, unfortunately, there have been no major breakthroughs (eg, a drug that can reverse kidney damage, or completely prevent rejection of kidney transplant). If there is a major breakthrough, be assured it will be introduced immediately. Many of the new innovations in dialysis are expensive and there has to be good research-based evidence that they are beneficial before they are used.

If a new discovery is made that is shown to benefit kidney patients, will it definitely be used? What if it is expensive? My unit always seems to be cutting corners to save money.

Most health care professionals are concerned with providing the best available treatments for their patients. The Renal Association produces guidelines for the treatment of adults with kidney failure, and these should help to ensure that the best treatments are used for all patients with kidney disease in the UK. For example, guidelines produced in 1997 state that 85% of all dialysis patients should have their anaemia treated so that their haemoglobin is more than 10g/dl. So, unless treatments are extremely expensive, there are mechanisms in place that will encourage doctors to use new treatments.

Unfortunately, there is no routine checking of renal units to make sure all these good things happen. There should be. There are also no sanctions against units that do not abide by these standards or use the best treatments. There should be these too.

The government has an agency called the National Institute for Clinical Excellence (NICE), whose role is to assess research based evidence and make recommendations for practice in the UK. At the time of publication, NICE had not assessed any treatments for kidney disease but there are plans to carry some out. So we cannot be sure at present that all discoveries are being passed on to your unit, or to you.

My husband is 32 years old and has been told he has IgA nephropathy. It will cause kidney failure but it is in quite an early stage. I have talked this through with him and we are keen to help research into a cure. But there are no studies being done on IgA nephropathy at our unit just now. So, what can we do to help?

There are a few research studies taking place that look into the causes and progression of kidney failure. These studies usually concern one cause of kidney failure (such as IgA nephropathy). And so, if you wanted to be involved, you would have to have the disease that was being studied. You should ask your doctor if there is any research about your disease going on in another unit.

There is little research going on into a cure for kidney failure. Once your kidneys have become damaged there is currently no way of reversing that damage, in most patients. Realistically, the best you can expect is that the progression of the disease can be halted, or at least slowed down. However, you should not be dissuaded from taking part in research that might help slow down the disease or otherwise improve your husband's life. Again ask your consultant about research going on, if necessary in other units, about 'progression'. This is the name we use for studies about the slowing down of kidney failure. There may be other research studies into the role of heart disease, exercise, high blood pressure control or genetics.

I have kidney failure and am keen to see that something good comes of this. On my death, I'd like to donate my kidneys for medical research. Is there a bank of kidneys of the people who have died of kidney failure, like the brain bank for people of have died of Alzheimer's disease? Can researchers learn from these organs?

There is currently no such bank in the UK. In fact, by looking at a dead person's kidney, it is difficult to gain a great deal of insight into the causes of kidney disease, what makes it get worse, or how it can be treated. Even though your kidneys are unlikely to be useful, however, it is possible that other organs will be – for example, your corneas, bones, heart valves and skin. So if you want to donate organs after your death, you should tell your relatives, and your doctor and nurse. In some areas of the country, the transplant co-ordinators can help to arrange the retrieval of some of your organs for research. It may be worth discussing it with them.

I am on haemodialysis and would like to take part in research to help the next generation of patients. There does not seem to be much going on in our unit. What can I do?

First talk to your nurse and doctor. If they are unable to help, find out the name of the research nurse who works in your unit, and phone or write to him or her. You could also contact the clinical director (senior consultant) who will be aware of all the research that is taking part in your unit.

You could also contact other large renal units in your area where there may be more research going on.

Where can I get up-to-date, accurate information on research into kidney failure?

A number of medical journals and magazines specialise in kidney disease, but these are written by experts for experts, and can be difficult to read. The best places are often on the Internet. Here are the addresses of some websites that have advice and information and links to other good sites.

- www.kidneywise.com

- www.nkrf.org.uk

- www.kidney.org.uk

- www.kidneypatientguide.org.uk.

If you are interested in specific projects or hospital activities try the website for the study or for your local hospital. For example: www.kingshealth.com (for King's College Hospital, London) and www.uhl-tr.nhs.uk (for Leicester).

Where does the funding for medical research into kidney failure come from?

Funding for medical research in the UK comes from anywhere researchers can the find money! Important sources of funding include the NHS Research and Development Fund, the Wellcome Trust and the Medical Research Council. Most pharmaceutical companies support or sponsor a number of research projects. Some big companies fund large research projects as well as trials of their own drugs. Specific kidney failure studies can get sponsorship through the National Kidney Research Fund (NKRF) and various other kidney related charities.

Ethics and drug trials

What processes must a drug for kidney failure go through before it becomes available for general use?

All drugs licensed for use in humans in the UK have to be studied thoroughly for their safety before they can be prescribed. We also have to make sure they work. This is usually done in animals first. Once the drug has been developed in the laboratory, it will go through four phases of human trial.

- **Phase 1:** Small, increasing doses of the drug are given for the first time to humans. Volunteers are paid, and are usually young healthy men. Women of childbearing age are usually excluded from this phase of studies – to avoid the risk of exposing an unborn baby to new drugs, in the very early stages of pregnancy. The main aim of this phase is to assess how the body copes with the drug – ie, whether it is safe, not whether it works.

- **Phase 2:** The drug is given for the first time to patients who need it, enabling the correct dose of the drug to be determined.

- **Phase 3:** These studies involve large numbers of patients and are normally carried out worldwide. The drug has to be proven to be as good as, or better than, existing drugs. If this is so, the company that makes the drug can apply for a licence to sell the drug.

- **Phase 4:** These trials look at the usefulness of the drug in particular groups of patients. They occur once the drug has been licensed, to broaden the use of the drug. An example might be testing a drug that has been proven to be useful used in the general population, on people with renal disease – eg, a new blood pressure tablet on patients with kidney failure.

How can I be sure a drug trial will be safe if I agree to take part?

All studies involving patients must be approved by a Local Research Ethical Committee (LREC). This committee will make sure the trial is worthwhile, and as safe as possible. The committee is made up of doctors and members of the public who are not connected to the trial in any way. If a study is taking place in more than five hospitals in the UK, approval will have to be gained from the Multicentre Research Ethics Committee (MREC). You can find out more about MREC and the ethics of medical research via the Internet on www.mrec.co.uk

I've been asked to take part in a study of a new PD fluid. What questions should I ask the doctor before I agree to take part in a study? I want to help other people but I am worried about my health.

You are under no obligation to take part in research, although it is great if you do. You should be sure the nurse or doctor running the study answers the following questions:

- What is the background to the study, and why is it being done?
- What will you have to do?
- How long will the study last?
- What are the potential side effects of the study?
- Can you withdraw at any time?
- Will information from the study be kept confidential?
- Will information be used to write articles for the medical press and could this information get into the national press?
- Will any side effects of the drugs in the trials be reported to the Committee for the Safety of Medicines (CSM)?
- Can you get compensation for any expenses you may have?

For example, taxi fares or petrol and parking for extra trips to hospital required by the study.

- Has the study been approved by the Local Research Ethics Committee or the Multicentre Research Ethics Committee?

- If the trial is being sponsored by a drug company, have they signed up to compensation guidelines and do they have insurance against any problems that could occur?

- Have you been told that the company sponsoring the study will have access to your medical records to verify results and examinations?

- Will your future treatment be affected by whether or not you take part in the study?

After consenting to the study you will be seen frequently by members of staff from the research team (usually nurses) for the duration of the study. You should be given clear instructions as to who you should contact if you have any questions during the time of the study. Some drug trials will include a 24-hour helpline.

I've agreed to take part in a study about a new blood pressure drug. Will I get paid? Could I come to any harm?

It is not usual for people taking part in drug trials, other than phase 1 trials, to be paid. You should expect to be paid for travel expenses. You may get a small sum of money if the study is undertaken by a pharmaceutical (drug) company, and if it involves some inconvenience to you (such as overnight stays in hospital).

Yes, you could come to some harm. But, the risks should be low, especially if the questions above have been answered to your satisfaction. Don't be pressurised into taking part. You should be given the opportunity to take a written information sheet away with you; and also be given as much time as you need (at least 24 hours) before making a decision about taking part in the study. Take your time before you 'sign on the dotted line'. Maybe speak to other patients already in the study. How are they feeling?

My husband is taking part in a study that is testing a new treatment for kidney failure. We have been told he may have the proper drug or the placebo – they won't say which. What is the placebo? Why can't we know which he is having? What happens if there is a problem with the drug (or the placebo for that matter)?

Placebo drugs are tablets (or injections) that look exactly the same as the drug that is being tested but have no effect on the body. They are dummy pills or injections. The idea of the placebo is quite simple. When testing a new drug (say a headache tablet), it is important to be sure the drug cured the headache, and not the meeting with the doctor or nurse. A study that involves a placebo is called a 'placebo-controlled study'.

So, if there was a trial for a headache pill, some people would be given the real pill and others the dummy. Both groups would be seen by health professionals. If the headaches got better in both groups, it is likely the meeting with the doctors and nurses was in part responsible for curing the headache. But if the people on the real pill get better, and those on the dummy do not, you can be sure the real pill has had an effect.

Using a placebo is usually done together with 'double blinding' (also called double masking). This means the researchers and the patients do not know whether the patient is on the real or dummy tablet. In this way, the researcher cannot influence the outcome of the study to prove that the real tablet works. However, in the case of an emergency – say an allergic reaction to the drug (or the placebo) – the researcher can find out which tablet your husband was on, and he can be taken out of the study.

My husband has been on a trial for a new drug. It seems to be making him feel better on dialysis. The trial has now stopped. Can he continue the drug?

First of all, you need to check that he had the drug rather than the placebo (if it was a placebo-controlled study). Assuming he was taking the drug, if the trial was a phase 3 or 4 one (see above), he can probably still take it. This is because at this point the company who make the drug will have obtained a licence for it. In earlier phases of a trial for a new drug, if it appears that the drug is considerably better than the usual drug, then your doctor may be able to get it for your husband on compassionate grounds. You should discuss this with your study nurse or doctor.

My elderly mother, a haemodialysis patient, is in a drug trial. Why does she have to make so many visits to the hospital? Why not just see them once at the end? She is coming up three times a week for dialysis anyway.

People on drug trials need careful monitoring. The reasons for this include:

(i)   making sure that the medication under trial is doing what it is supposed to do;
(ii) making sure that any known side effects of the drug are monitored regularly;
(iii) looking out for new side effects of the drug;
(iv) ensuring that patients are taking the drug as prescribed.

If your mother was not seen until the end of the trial then many of these things might go unnoticed and this could be dangerous. There may be a good reason why she cannot be seen by the research nurse on the same day that she has dialysis. If the frequent trips are becoming a burden on your mother, she should discuss this with the nurse and perhaps consider withdrawing from the study.

My wife is in a trial of a new drug for dialysis patients. What happens if the drug given in a trial turns out to be harmful?

It is unlikely that any drug that is being studied on dialysis patients will be harmful – partly as it should have been tried out in normal humans first. However, safety measures are set up in all research studies. For example, all trials must report any unusual side effect that occurs during the study. If the side effect happens often, then the trial safety committee (who are not part of the trial team) will call for the study to be stopped.

Before any study starts, the company producing a new drug should sign an indemnity (insurance) document with the hospital. This document makes sure that in the unlikely event of a patient being harmed by the drug, the company will compensate the patient and their family. The content of the indemnity document is the same throughout the UK. You should ask to see the evidence that the trial has such an insurance scheme – not all do.

Getting involved and lobbying

Where can I get information on kidney failure?

Most renal units have a Kidney Patient Association. This is a charitable support group, formed by kidney patients, for kidney patients and their relatives. Most local associations are affiliated to a national kidney charity, the National Kidney Federation (NKF). They have a helpline (see Appendix 2). Your kidney consultant should be able to give you information about your condition, and the nurses should be able to answer questions related to dialysis. Other sources of information include the following.

(i)   Most renal units have a range of free leaflets available about kidney failure and its treatment.

(ii) The National Kidney Research Fund (NKRF) has a helpline (see Appendix 2). This helpline offers a self-assessment test kit to detect early signs of kidney disease. It is open every day of the year including Christmas and bank holidays.

(iii) The NKF also has a regular magazine (*Kidney Life*) for kidney patients, and publishes booklets on many aspects of kidney failure, haemodialysis, PD, etc. You can write and ask for a list.

(iv) Your renal unit may run pre-dialysis education sessions.

(v)   There are several good books available (apart from this one!). *Kidney Failure Explained*, by the same authors of this book, contains more medical information. Or you could look at Professor Stewart Cameron's in-depth book *Kidney Failure, The Facts*. You can order either book from your bookshop. The Coventry Renal Unit produces a free book, *Help I've Got Kidney Failure*. You can write to Dr Higgins' secretary, enclosing a large stamped addressed envelope, for a copy. The address is Renal Unit, Walsgrave Hospital, Coventry CV2 2DX.

(vi) There is an increasing number of useful websites – see Appendix 3 for a list.

(vii) Suppliers of dialysis equipment, such as Baxter, produce booklets on treatment options.

I am so angry about the lack of facilities for haemodialysis in my hospital. I felt forced to go on PD as I would have to wait ages for a haemodialysis slot. What can I do about it?

Ideally, patients should be able to decide which treatment will best suit their lives, if all the options are medically equivalent. However, many units are so short of resources and nursing staff, that haemodialysis is not offered as a first choice of treatment. Those patients offered haemodialysis tend to be those for whom PD is not medically advisable or possible. Where resources are stretched, patients may be offered twice-weekly haemodialysis. This is known to be less effective for health and well-being than treatment three times a week. You should remember that for a number of patients, PD is actually the most suitable treatment, providing a flexible and independent way of dialysing.

If you want hospital haemodialysis, you should let your consultant know. If you are told that lack of resources is the problem, you could join a local or national Patients' Association to get involved in the political debate over lack of funding. You could write to your MP and explain the position. Get him or her to take an interest. Kidney patients need to be heard if they are to get the funding that is needed.

I'm a carer for my father, a haemodialysis patient. I'd like to get involved in political lobbying, as I have been appalled by the quality of his care. It's not the doctors and nurses, they are trying their best. They just have inadequate facilities. What can I do?

Publicity is a powerful tool. Why not write to your local paper with the story? The best organisation to join is the National Kidney Federation (NKF), who speak for all kidney patients, and have links with the Renal All-Party Group, a group of MPs who fight for resources for kidney patients.

I am on PD and have lost my job. I'm keen to do something constructive for the unit, or start up a club for patients. Can you advise?

If there is no Patients' Association in your area, it would be an excellent idea to start one. You could also talk to your unit, and find out if there are any particular projects for which money is needed. These might be for equipment to improve the comfort and well-being of patients and carers. It is a good idea to approach local firms who may be willing to provide sponsorship for events to raise money. The well-being of patients and carers can also be improved through psychological support, which covers everything from meeting at a coffee morning to seeing a counsellor. So, yes you could set up a club for patients. It is all about confidence, self-esteem and morale. It certainly helps both patients and carers to meet others in the same position, and to spark ideas off each other.

If you have lost your job, it is good for you to realise that you could now be doing something even more worthwhile with your time.

What can I do to help my Renal Unit? There never seem to be enough haemodialysis machines. Should I buy one?

In the past, it was helpful for patients to raise money for your unit to buy haemodialysis machines. They are very expensive and renal units never have enough. However, these days buying a machine is not that helpful. There are many added costs, such as service contracts, nursing support and disposable equipment that are needed to keep the machine running. The technology goes out of date very quickly, requiring new machines all the time. The biggest problem in most renal units is a lack of nurses to operate the machines. Recruitment of new nurses is a national problem that cannot be easily fixed by raising money.

If you want to buy an object that will help a renal unit (and may last quite a while), you could consider buying an intravenous pump, or a blood pressure machine.

I'm retired and on PD, so I have a lot of time. What else can I do to help, financially or otherwise?

Raising money is always helpful and can be used for patient welfare. For example, the renal unit might need more televisions, comfortable chairs or a trip away for patients and their carers. But what is also of use is to be an active member of the KPA to help solve some of the bigger issues. You may need to become more outspoken to publicise the problems.

Writing to or visiting your MP at his/her local surgery may help considerably. Not all politicians are aware of the major problems in British kidney medicine. Keep visiting them.

Sound bites such as 'patients are dying day in, day out, through lack of dialysis capability' are true, and you should use them. But it is important, before you go, to make sure you know the local and national position on renal services, and have the data with you, rather than come out with a series of sound bites.

There is now a Parliamentary All-Party Group in Kidney Medicine. Make sure your MP is aware of that group. Try to get him or her to join the group.

If you have the time, and want to operate at a national level, join the NKF. Whatever you do, no matter how small, we are sure it will be helpful to our cause . . . you.

Appendix 1
Summary of normal and target blood test results for patients on dialysis

	Substance	Relevance
Dialysable substances	Sodium	Fluid balance
	Potassium	Heart health
	Glucose	Blood sugar
	Creatinine	Toxin clearance
	Urea	Toxin clearance
	Bicarbonate	Acid balance
	Calcium	Bone health
	Phosphate	Bone health
Non-dialysable substances	Albumin	Nutritional status
	Bilirubin	Liver function
	AST	Liver function
	Alk. phos.	Liver function
	GammaGT	Liver function
Other (non-dialysable) substances	Haemoglobin	Blood health
	Ferritin	Iron in blood
	Parathyroid hormone	Bone health

How do your test results compare? Although your hospital may use slightly different figures, they should be similar to those given here. If any of your figures do not seem to be on target, find out why.

Normal level	Target level	Units
136–144	Normal	mcmol/l
3.7–5.0	Normal	mcmol/l
3.0–7.8	Normal	mcmol/l
70–120	Less than 800	mcmol/l
3.7–8.1	Less than 25	mcmol/l
21–29	High-normal (26–29)	mcmol/l
2.2–2.6	High-normal (2.5–2.6)	mcmol/l
0.8–1.4	Less than 1.8	mcmol/l
34–48	Normal	g/l
4–25	Normal	mmol/l
8–40	Normal	iu/l
30–120	Normal	iu/l
10–70	Normal	iu/l
11.7–18	10–12	g/dl
15–350	More than 200	mcg/l
1.1–4.2	Less than 15	pmol/l

(This table first appeared in *Kidney Failure Explained*, by Andy Stein and Janet Wild, Class Publishing.)

Appendix 2
Useful Addresses

Please note that addresses
change from time to time.

**Access to Communication
and Technology**
Oak Tree Lane Centre
Oak Tree Lane
Selly Oak
Birmingham B29 6JA
Tel: 0121 627 8235
Fax: 0121 627 8210
*NHS centre offering a wide
range of services throughout the
UK to assist people of any age
with disabilities, including
assessment and rehabilitation,
home equipment loan service,
artificial limbs, electrical
appliances and training by
professionals.*

Age Concern England
Astral House
1268 London Road
London SW16 4ER
Tel: 020 8679 8000
Fax: 020 8766 7211
Helpline: 0800 009 966
Website: www.ace.org.uk
*Researches into the needs of
older people and is involved in
policy making. Publishes many
books and has useful fact sheets
on a wide range of issues from
benefits to care, and provides
services via local branches.*

**Action on Smoking and Health
(ASH)**
102 Clifton Street
London EC2A 4HW
Tel: 020 7739 5902
Fax: 020 7613 0531
Helpline: 0800 169 0169
Website: www.ash.org.uk
*Information on how smoking
affects medical conditions.*

British Association of Counselling
1 Regent Place
Rugby
Warwickshire CV21 2PJ
Tel: 08788 550 899
Fax: 0870 443 5161
Website: www.counselling.co.uk
Will give advice about counselling services in your area. Send s.a.e. for information and publications list.

British Heart Foundation (BHF)
14 Fitzhardinge Street
London W1H 6DH
Tel: 020 7935 0185
Fax: 020 7486 5820
Website: www.bhs.org.uk
Funds research into heart disease. Provides help and advice.

British Kidney Patient Association
Bordon
Hampshire GU35 9JZ
Tel: 01420 472 021
Fax: 01420 4725 831
Website: www.bkpa.org.uk
Provides information and advice to people with kidney illnesses throughout the UK. Grants available.

Cancerlink
Macmillan Cancer Relief
89 Albert Embankment
London SE1 7UQ
Tel: 020 7840 7840
Fax: 020 7840 7841
Helpline: 0808 808 0000
Website: www.cancerlink.org
Helps cancer patients, families and carers with practical and emotional support.

Carers' National Association
20–25 Glasshouse Yard
London EC1A 4JT
Tel: 020 7490 8818
Fax: 020 7490 8824
Helpline: 0808 808 7777
Website: www.carers.demon.co.uk
Offers information and support to all people who have to care for others due to medical or other problems.

Carers Scotland
91 Mitchell Street
Glasgow G1 3LN
Tel: 0141 221 9141
Fax: 0141 221 9140
Helpline: 0808 808 7777
Offers information and support to all people who have to care for others due to medical or other problems.

Contact a Family
209–211 City Road
London EC1V 1JN
Tel: 020 7608 8701
Fax: 020 7608 8701
Helpline: 0808 808 3555
Website: www.cafamily.org.uk
Helpline for parents of children with special needs. Also has comprehensive information of rare syndromes affecting people of all ages. Loose leaf directory available to buy.

Counsel & Care
Lower Ground Floor
Twyman House
16 Bonny Street
London NW1 9PG
Tel: 020 7485 1566
Fax: 020 7267 6877
Helpline: 0845 300 7585
Website:
www.counselandcare.org.uk
Offers information to the elderly on welfare rights, benefits, community care, helps with choice of residential homes, including inspection and registration of units. Some grants available.

Crossroads Association
10 Regent Place
Rugby
Warwicks CV21 2PN
Tel: 01788 573 653
Fax: 01788 565 498
Website: www.crossroads.org.uk
Supports and delivers high quality services for carers and people with care needs via its local branches.

Crossroads Scotland
Care Attendant Schemes
24 George Square
Glasgow G2 1EG
Tel: 0141 226 3793
Fax: 0141 221 7130
Website:
www.crossroadsscot.fsnet.co.uk
Information leaflets and support for carers within own homes, for any age, disability and sickness. Local branches.

Cruse
126 Sheen Road
Richmond
Surrey TW9 1UR
Tel: 020 8940 4818
Fax: 020 8940 7638
Helpline: 0870 167 1677
Website: www.
crusebereavementcare.org.uk
Offers information, sells literature and has local branches which can provide one-to-one bereavement counselling.

Department of Health
Richmond House
79 Whitehall
London SW1A 2NS
Tel: 020 7210 4850
Website: www.
open.gov.uk/doh/dhhome.htm
*Government department
involved with policy making and
health service issues.*

**Department of Work
and Pensions**
Disability Benefit Centre
Olympic House
Olympic Way
Wembley
Middlesex HA9 0DL
Tel: 020 8795 8400
Helpline: 0800 88 22 00
*Government information service
offering advice on benefits for
people with disabilities and
their carers.*

Depression Alliance
35 Westminster Bridge Road
London SE1 7JB
Tel: 020 7633 9929
Fax: 020 7633 0559
Website:
www.depressionalliance.org
*Offers support and understand-
ing to anyone affected by depression, and relatives who want
help. Has a network of self help
groups, correspondence schemes
and a range of literature. Send
s.a.e. for information.*

Diabetes UK
10 Queen Anne Street
London W1G 9LH
Tel: 020 7323 1531
Fax: 020 7637 3644
Helpline: 020 7636 6112
Website: www.diabetes.org.uk
*Provides advice and
information on diabetes; has
local support groups.*

Disability Scotland
Princes House
5 Shandwick Place
Edinburgh EH2 4RG
Tel: 0131 339 8632
Fax: 0131 339 5168
Website: www.dis-scot.gcal.ac.uk

**Disability Wales/Anabledd
Cymru**
Llys Ilfor
Crescent Road
Caerphilly
Mid Glamorgan CF83 1XL
Tel: 029 2088 7325
Fax: 029 2088 8702
e-mail: info@dwac.demon.co.uk

Disabled Living Foundation
380–384 Harrow Road
London W9 2HU
Helpline: 0845 130 9177
Tel: 020 7289 6111
Fax: 020 7266 2922
Website: www.dlf.org.uk
*Provides information on all
kinds of equipment for people
with special needs.*

DVLA (Drivers and Vehicles Licensing Authority)
Medical Branch
Longview Road
Morriston
Swansea SA99 1TU
Tel: 01792 772151
Fax: 01792 783779
Helpline: 0870 6000301
Website: www.dvla.gov.uk
Government office providing advice for drivers with special needs.

Employment Opportunities for People with Disabilities
123 Minories
London EC3N 1NT
Tel: 020 7481 2727
Fax: 020 7481 9797
Website:
www.opportunities.org.uk

Family Fund
PO Box 50
York YO1 2XZ
Tel: 01904 621 115
Fax: 01904 652 625
Provides grants, household equipment and repairs

Family Holiday Association
2nd Floor Rear
16 Mortimer Street
London W1M 7RD
Tel: 020 7436 3304
Fax: 020 7436 3302
Website: www.fhaonnline.org.uk
Free Prescriptions Advice Line
Tel: 0800 9177 711
(Mon–Fri 8am–6pm;
Sat & Sun 10am–4pm)
Advice on entitlement to free prescriptions, dental and optical care.

Holiday Care
Imperial Buildings, 2nd Floor
Victoria Road
Horley
Surrey
RH6 7PZ
Tel: 01293 774 535
Fax: 01293 784 647
Information and advice about holidays, travel or respite care for older or disabled people and carers.

Impotence Association
P O Box 10296
London SW17 9WH
Website: www.impotence.org.uk
Offers help and advice on sexual problems.

Institute for Complementary Medicine
PO Box 194
London SE16 7QZ
Tel: 020 7237 5165
Fax: 020 7237 5175
Website: www.icmedicine.co.uk
Umbrella group for complementary medicine organisations.

Kidney Cancer UK
11 Hathaway Road
Tile Hill Village
Coventry CV4 9HW
Tel: 02476 470 584
Fax: 02476 470 584
Website: kcuk.org
Information and support for people with kidney cancer and their carers.
Chat room available via the website.

Medic-Alert Foundation
1 Bridge Wharf
156 Caledonian Road
London N1 9UU
Tel: 020 7833 3034
Fax: 020 2213 5653
e-mail: info@medicalert.co.uk
Offers selection of jewellery with internationally recognised medical symbol: 24-hour emergency phoneline.

MIND (National Association for Mental Health)
Granta House
15–19 Broadway
Stratford
London E15 4BQ
Tel: 020 8519 2122
Fax: 020 8522 1725
Helpline: 0845 766 0163
Website: www.mind.org.uk
Mental health organisation working for a better life for everyone experiencing mental distress. Has information and offers support via local branches.

Motability
Goodman House
Station Approach
Harlow
Essex CM20 2ET
Tel: 01279 635666
Fax: 01279 632000
Advice and help about cars, scooters and wheelchairs for disabled people.

National Kidney Federation
6 Stanley Street
Worksop
Notts S81 7HX
Tel: 01909 487 795
Fax: 01909 481 723
Helpline: 0845 601 0209
E-mail: nkf@kidney.org.uk
Website: www.kidney.org.uk
Aims to promote, throughout the United Kingdom, the welfare of people suffering from kidney failure and those relatives and friends who care for them.

National Kidney Research Fund
King's Chambers
Priestgate
Peterborough PE1 1FG
Tel: 01733 704 650
Fax: 01733 704 692
Helpline: 0845 300 1499
E-mail: enquiries@nkrf.org.uk
Website: www.nkrf.org.uk
Funds research into kidney disease, its causes and treatment. Also working towards raising awareness of kidney disease.

Patients Association
PO Box 935
Harrow
Middlesex HA1 3YJ
Tel: 020 8423 9111
Fax: 020 8423 9119
Helpline: 0845 608 4455
Website: www.patients-association.com
Provides advice on patients' rights.

Registered Nursing Homes Association
Calthorpe House
Hagley Road
Edgbaston
Birmingham B16 8QY
Tel: 0121 454 2511
Fax: 0121 454 9032
Website: www.rnha.co.uk
Information about registered nursing homes in your area.

Relate
Herbert Gray College
Little Church Street
Rugby
Warwickshire CV21 3AP
Tel: 01788 573 241
Fax: 01788 535 007
Helpline: 09069 123 715
Website: www.relate.org.uk
Formerly the Marriage Guidance Council. Offers relationship counselling via local branches.

SPOD
286 Camden Road
London N& 0BJ
Tel: 020 7607 8851
Fax: 020 7700 0236
*Association to aid the sexual
and personal relationships of
disabled people.*

Terrence Higgins Trust
52–54 Gray's Inn Road
London WC1X 8JU
Tel: 020 7831 0330
Website: www.tht.org.uk
*Provides information, support
and advice relating to HIV and
AIDS. Now has branches in
major cities throughout the UK –
see website for details.*

**United Kingdom Register
of Counsellors**
P O Box 1050
Rugby
Warwickshire CV21 2HZ
Tel: 0870 443 5232
Fax: 0870 443 5161
*Part of British Association of
Counselling and Psychotherapy.
Regulatory body which provides
details of registered counsellors
who offer safe and accountable
practice.*

Winged Fellowship Trust
Angel House
20/32 Pentonville Road
London N1 9XD
Tel: 020 7833 2594
Fax: 020 7278 0370
Website: www.wft.org.uk
*Provides holidays and respite
care for disabled people and
their carers.*

Appendix 3
Resources

Websites

http://web.bma.org.uk/transplant.nsf
The transplant partnership.

http://www.bmj.com
The British Medical Journal *website.*

http://www.eurodial.org/
The international dialysis organisation dedicated to the care and mobility of dialysis patients.

http://www.fastuk.org
A forum for information and exchange of ideas for all those involved in the development of assistive technology, or its use.

http://www.globaldialysis.com
Gives details of holidays and travel information for dialysis patients.

http://www.ikidney.com
A worldwide kidney disease community.

http://www.kidney.org
The website of the National Kidney Federation in the USA.

http://www.kidney.org.uk
The website of the National Kidney Federation of the UK.

http://www.kidneydirections.com
Information for kidney patients and suggestions for ways to plan treatment.

http://www.kidneypatientguide.org.uk
Information for patients with kidney failure and those who care for them.

http://www.kidneywise.com
Help advice and support for those affected by kidney failure.

http://www.mrec.co.uk
Medical Research Council website – gives information about research in progress and the rights of participating patients.

http://www.nephronline.org
Kidney medicine at your fingertips!

http://news.bbc.co.uk
Health-related news from the BBC.

http://www.nhsdirect.nhs.uk
The NHS Direct website – your gateway to health information on the Internet.

http://www.nhsorgandonor.net
NHS organ donor website.

http://www.nlm.nih.gov
The United States National Library of Medicine.

http://www.renalnet.org
Renalnet – the kidney information clearing house.

http://www.renalreg.com
The renal registry of the UK – responsible for the collection and analysis of data relating to the numbers, treatment and outcomes of patients with kidney failure..

http://www.s4lk.co.uk/
Strength for living – kidney disease. Information about anaemia in kidney failure.

http://www.surgerydoor.co.uk
A health website for the UK.

http://tjktsc.tripod.com
Jewish kidney and transplant support centre.

http://www.uktransplant.org.uk
The UK Transplant Support Service Authority website.

Further reading

Stewart Cameron, *Kidney Failure: the facts*. Oxford Paperbacks.

Stewart Cameron, *History of the Treatment of Kidney Failure by Dialysis*. Oxford University Press.

Kevin Kendrick and Simon Robinson, *Living Wills*. Age Concern Books.

Lawrence Keogh and Rashmi Soni, *Food for Life*. Class Publishing.

Norman Levinski, *Ethics and the Kidney*. Oxford University Press.

Jeremy Levy, Julie Morgan and Edwina Brown, *Oxford Handbook of Dialysis*. Oxford University Press.

Hannah McGee and Clare Bradley, *Quality of Life Following Renal Failure*. Harwood Academic.

Toni Smith and Nicky Thomas, *Renal Nursing*. Balliere Tindall.

Peter Sonksen, Charles Fox and Sue Judd, *Diabetes: The At Your Fingertips Guide*. Class Publishing.

Andy Stein and Janet Wild, *Kidney Failure Explained*. Class Publishing.

Julian Tudor Hart and Tom Fahey, *High Blood Pressure: The At Your Fingertips Guide*. Class Publishing.

Jacob van Noordwijk, *Dialysing for Life*. Kluwer Academic Publishers.

Index

and pregnancy 211
research into levels 258
test 26–7, 73–4, 78, 140
very high level 67–8, 80–1
cross-matching
blood groups 130, 137–8
kidneys for transplant 129
tissue types 130–2, 138
Crossroads Care 231
CT *see* computerised tomography
(CT) scan
Customs and Excise 174, 180–1
CVP *see* central venous pressure
cyclophosphamide 64
cyclosporin 145, 164, 165–6, 167
during breastfeeding 214
cystoscopy 77, 82
cysts 15, 19–20, 48
see also polycystic disease
cytomegalovirus (CMV) 133, 146

dairy produce 46, 59, 60
day surgery 83
DDD *see* dense deposit disease
death 11, 42, 66, 89, 251–4
of donors 126
see also life expectancy;
spiritual needs
dehydration 50, 58
dementia 252
denial of one's situation 219
dense deposit disease (DDD) 31
dental problems *see* teeth
depression 207, 218, 220–3
see also psychological
problems
deterioration of kidneys 18, 28–9
diabetes 6–7, 15, 20–1
access problems 122
age factor 16
cardiac catheter test 134

caused by immunosuppressants
165–7
choice of fistula site 116
diabetic kidney disease 30–1
in donors 155
'double transplants' 149–50
factor in choice of treatment 92
factor in survival *35*
leg ulcers 229
and PD as treatment option 106
in prospective donors 155
race risk 10, 20
and transplants 32, 70–1
diagnosis 12, 41, 48, 75
by ultrasound scan 85, 86
dialysis 4, 12–13
access sites 112–13
age factor 10, 33–7
and anaemia 54
before transplant 125
and calcium levels 61–2
choice of type 70, 91–2, 122,
194–5
comparing UK with rest of
Europe 37–9, *38*
cost 98–9, 123
and creatinine levels 12, 67–8,
74, 78–9, 80
delaying need for 18–19
diet while waiting to start 47
and employment 189
for ESRF 67
fluid *see main heading* fluid
'going flat' 120
insufficient 45
limitations of treatment 92
machines 91, 96, 103, 112–13
how they work 117, 118–19,
119
and sexual activity 209
main reasons for starting 11–12

vitamin D 46, 60, 62, 63
Voltarol 65
vomiting 58, 120, 165, 168

waiting list for transplant 125–6,
    132–5
  after failed transplant 142–3
  after years of dialysis 154
  finding the recipient 135–6, 151
  removal from list 135
waiting for tests 86
warfarin 117
waste products 3–5, *3*, 7, 120
  dangerously high level 12, 26, 42
  in haemodialysis dialysis
      machine *119*
  liver function 80
water
  abroad 180, 181
  dangerously high level 12
  excess 1, *3*, 4, 5, 7, 120
  means of losing 55–6
  and PD fluid 105
  sucked from blood 91
  tablets 121
  see also fluid balance
water tablets *see* diuretics
weakness feeling 47, 58, 109

weather and urine excretion 5
weight problems 6, 10, 22, 185–6
  and haemodialysis 32–3
  loss 46, 58, 123, 148
  obesity of donors 155
  slimming 185–6
  sudden increase 56, 168
welfare *see* benefits; grants; help,
    financial
Welfare Rights Advice Centre 239
wheezing 145
wills 244
work *see* employment

X-ray 134, 156, *see also* angio-
    gram; computerised
    tomography (CT) scan;
    intrvenous pyelogram;
    nephrostomy; nuclear
    medicine scan; ultrasound
    scan
xenotransplantation 150

young people *see* age, young
    people

Zestril 65

Have you found **Kidney Dialysis and Transplants – the 'at your fingertips' guide** practical and useful? If so, you may be interested in other books from Class Publishing.

Kidney Failure Explained
NEW SECOND EDITION! £14.99
Dr Andy Stein and Janet Wild
The complete and updated reference manual for people suffering from kidney failure, which tells you everything you need to know about the condition.
This is a book for anyone with kidney problems, their families and friends and those who look after the needs of people with a kidney condition, including GP's, practice nurses and specialist nurses.

> 'I believe this excellent book should be read by every kidney patient and their family. I can recommend it without hesitation.'
> *Austin Donohoe, Chairman, National Kidney Federation*

Heart health – the 'at your fingertips' guide
Dr Graham Jackson £14.99
This practical handbook, written by a leading cardiologist, answers all your questions about heart conditions.

> 'Contains the answers the doctor wishes he had given if only he'd had the time'
> *Dr Thomas Stuttaford, The Times*

High blood pressure - the 'at your fingertips' guide
Dr Julian Tudor Hart with Dr Tom Fahey
£14.99
The authors use all their years of experience as blood pressure experts to answer your questions on high blood pressure.

> 'Readable and comprehensive information.'
> *Dr Sylvia McLaughlan, Director General, The Stoke Association*

Stop that heart attack!
SECOND EDITION! £14.99
Dr Derrick Cutting
The easy, drug-free and medically accurate way to cut your risk of having a heart attack dramatically.
Even if you already have heart disease, you can halt and even reverse its progress by following Dr Cutting's simple steps. Don't be a victim – take action NOW!

Diabetes - the 'at your fingertips' guide
FOURTH EDITION! £14.99
Professor Peter Sonksen,
Dr Charles Fox and Sister Sue Judd
461 questions on diabetes are answered clearly and accurately - the ideal reference book for everyone with diabetes.

Beating depression – the 'at your fingertips' guide
NEW! £14.99
Dr Stefan Cembrowicz and Dr Dorcas Kingham
This positive handbook, written by two medical experts, gives practical advice on overcoming depression and anxiety. It covers the different treatments available, and offers self-help techniques.

Dementia: Alzheimer's and other dementias – the 'at your fingertips' guide
NEW SECOND EDITION! £14.99
Harry Cayton, Dr Nori Graham and Dr James Warner
At last – a book that tells you everything you need to know about Alzheimer's and other dementias.

> 'An invaluable contribution to understanding all forms of dementia.'
> *Dr Jonathan Miller CBE, President of the Alzheimer's Disease Society*

PRIORITY ORDER FORM

Cut out or photocopy this form and send it (post free in the UK) to:

Class Publishing Priority Service　　　　**Tel: 01752 202301**
FREEPOST (PAM 6219)　　　　　　　　　**Fax: 01752 202333**
Plymouth PL6 7ZZ

Please send me urgently　　　　　　　　*Post included*
(*tick boxes below*)　　　　　　　　*price per copy (UK only)*

☐ **Kidney Dialysis and Transplants – the 'at your fingertips'
guide**　　　　　　　　　　　　　　　　　　　　£17.99
(ISBN 1 859590 46 2)

☐ **Kidney Failure Explained**　　　　　　　　　£17.99
(ISBN 1 859590 70 5)

☐ **Heart health – the 'at your fingertips' guide**　　£17.99
(ISBN 1 859590 09 8)

☐ **High blood pressure – the 'at your fingertips' guide**　£17.99
(ISBN 1 872362 81 8)

☐ **Stop that heart attack!**　　　　　　　　　　£17.99
(ISBN 1 859590 55 1)

☐ **Diabetes – the 'at your fingertips' guide**　　　£17.99
(ISBN 1 872362 79 6)

☐ **Beating depression – the 'at your fingertips' guide**　£17.99
(ISBN 1 859590 62 3)

☐ **Dementia: Alzheimer's and other dementias – the 'at your**　£17.99
fingertips' guide
(ISBN 1 859590 75 6)

TOTAL _____

Easy ways to pay

Cheque: I enclose a cheque payable to Class Publishing for £ _____

Credit card: Please debit my ☐ Access ☐ Visa ☐ Amex ☐ Switch

Number _____ Expiry date _____

Name _____

My address for delivery is _____

_____

Town _____ County _____ Postcode _____

Telephone number (in case of query) _____

Credit card billing address if different from above _____

_____

Town _____ County _____ Postcode _____

*Class Publishing's guarantee: remember that if, for any reason, you are not satisfied with these books, we will refund all
your money, without any questions asked. Prices and VAT rates may be altered for reasons beyond our control.*